LYME SAVVY

TREATMENT INSIGHTS FOR

LYME PATIENTS AND PRACTITIONERS

SHARON E. RAINEY AND
B. ROBERT MOZAYENI, M.D.

Books by Sharon E. Rainey

Making a Pearl from the Grit of Life

The Best Part of My Day Healing Journal

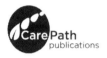

CAREPATH PUBLICATIONS

Copyright ©2016 by Sharon E. Rainey and B. Robert Mozayeni, M.D.

Lyme Savvy: Treatment Insights for Lyme Patients and Practitioners
by Sharon E. Rainey and B. Robert Mozayeni, M.D.

ISBN-13: 978-0983086826
ISBN-10: 0983086826

Cover by Look Design
CarePath Publications
1146-D Walker Road, Great Falls, VA 22066
www.carepathpublications.com
First printing December 2016

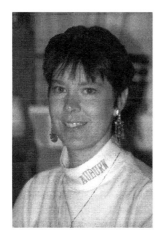 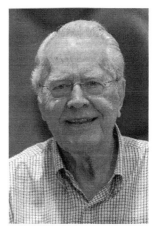

For Aunt Betty   **In Honor and Memory of Dad**

Nora Elizabeth Williams Brazelton   Earle Carter Williams

(1945 – 2002)   (1929 – 2016)

– SHARON RAINEY

To the patients, who through their suffering and perseverance,

touch the lives of those who witness their journey, and transform

themselves as much as they transform those who care for them.

– BOB MOZAYENI

Tues – 5:00 –
TR Thurs 3:00
Sat.

DIETARY RECOMMENDATIONS

SUGGESTIONS
FOR HOW TO
USE THIS BOOK

SHARON

We wrote this book with a dual purpose:

- We want chronically ill patients to have a book that offers validation and possible explanations for their conditions.
- We want physicians to have a book that helps them appreciate some of the medical and psychological issues faced by chronically ill patients and their care providers.

Because of this, sections of this book are easier to absorb than others. Our hope is each of you will read the parts first that "speak" to you; the ones you look at and say, "Oh, I want to know more about this." We do not expect this book to be read in the order the chapters appear. While it might be nice that way, it certainly is not necessary.

There might be sections that do not relate to you. Skip them if you like. Read them sometime later when you think they might apply.

Sometimes, it can be difficult to read a book with two separate authors' writing. We have tried to simplify this for the reader. You will notice on each page, when Dr. Mozayeni is "speaking," there are two vertical lines to the left of his text. When Sharon is "speaking," there is one vertical line. You might also notice that our name appears with those vertical lines at the beginning of almost each new subsection.

We hope there are sections in here you will want to share with your physicians, family, friends, and caregivers. Feel free to do so.

We do not want this to be a book you purchase and put on your bookshelf. **We want this book to be sitting on your nightstand with dog-eared pages, notes and highlights throughout.** We want this book to connect with you.

Whatever way works for you, please use this book as a guide, as validation, as an explanation, and as an offering to how you might heal from chronic illness.

SECTION ONE

VALIDATION & GOALS

"They need you to tell their stories so they are not forgotten or lost. Part of the healing comes from sharing their stories with you.

You will help others heal by sharing their stories."

– DEB JANSEN

FOREWARD

DR. MOZAYENI

I was first intellectually 'exposed' to Lyme during training at the Yale School-New Haven Hospital, during my residency in Internal Medicine and Fellowship Training in Rheumatology. It is not a coincidence the disease was first discovered by Rheumatologists and that the Lyme Clinic at Yale circa 1987 was run by the Rheumatology department.

This is because Lyme Disease is more of a disease with symptoms caused more by the host response, than by the microbe itself.

B burgdorferi, the bacterium, is not a flesh-eating microbe like some aggressive streptococcal infections that produces toxic flesh-dissolving enzymes or toxins, like Pertussis or Tetanus.

Lyme Disease has more to do with the type and intensity of the host response than the microbe itself. Lyme Disease is not an 'infectious disease' as much as it is a 'host-response' disease. And it is a host response to an array of microbes often seen together, referred to as 'co-infections.'

Therein lies the way we can understand the complexity and the confusion.

Fast forward to 2016, where I am now distinguishing in my medical practice between Lyme Disease (medical definition) and #Lyme Disease, the social networking definition. The social networking definition describes the problem and the need of patients. The medical definition is narrowly defined for research purposes and it does not translate into help for patients with myriad symptoms.

Because it is the host response that defines the disease, we have to expand our view of the host response to understand the #Lyme Disease.

The human social and medical host response to this germ, writ large, is marked by human endeavors, achievements, and conflicts; there is uncertainty plagued by policy maker dysfunction and huge variability in education. This awareness has the masses yearning to say whatever they want in a blog without regard for logic or scientific process. Yet, a new consciousness emerges from this maelstrom of mass Internet hysteria driven by desperation and the will to improve our lot individually and collectively.

Whom you choose to believe is irrelevant. New communication methods, genomics, 'big data', and computational methods have transformed how we think.

We now have a new way to think and innovate through a messy but awkwardly beautiful avenue to crowd-source solutions to problems, called the Internet.

In the world of the Internet, we can easily:

A. get information poisoning,

B. find the occasional golden nugget of information to guide our path, or

C. medically innovate our way to wellness.

As we wander through the Internet, we can also stick our fingers in the high voltage socket of human emotion and suffering.

If we carry desperation without love in our hearts, we can easily run into information, concepts, and people in which or whom we can readily take offense.

We can choose even, to watch TV networks that will feed our need to be offended in the way that we want to be offended.

Recognizing Lyme and #Lyme as a host-response disease, we could have predicted fully that we would have this controversy.

Over the years, I have learned something very important about chronic illness: as a disease process unfolds, it cascades in different directions and each cascade can then further cascade. As a result, one develops a complex set of inter-related symptoms.

Chronic illness is not about finding the singular cause, what is called in medicine, 'Achem's razor' but rather, chronic illness is caused by a wide range of possible contributing factors, to consider systematically and thoroughly with multiple iterations.

The root cause may have been something minor, like a non-pathogenic microbe inducing ever so slight an inflammatory response that later, cascaded into disease. To complicate it further, we have to appreciate that the majority of organisms discovered by science cannot be cultured, that we erroneously rely too heavily on measurements in blood, which is only one of the tissues of the body, telling us about disease in other tissues of the body.

And, finally, with all we can document in lab testing we have no conceivable way to know how much each finding contributes to each symptom. It becomes very easy for any chronic disease issue in medicine to be fraught with controversy.

In most matters, with controversy comes debate and dialogue. If both sides of a medical controversy approach the dialogue with love and compassion for those who suffer, then we can brainstorm a better solution.

But no, instead, people are able to find offense in a person, place or thing in advance of a meeting or dialogue. Because of this, offense is the posture before any conversation begins around a medical

controversy. This is also how our governments and po[...]
today - everyone has a partially formed but hardline opin[...]
thus, nobody can effectively lead.

My patients who heal, other physicians' patients who heal, and the doctors who heal them, work from the premise that healing is possible though it may be improbable. Hardliners in medical controversies think the world is binary, they are right or wrong, and that the odds of someone not healing means we should not try to heal them.

And, in a cost-constrained health care system where even at top medical centers a bone marrow transplant candidate gets only 20 minutes with their oncologist, we have created the most impersonal type of health care system we could have imagined - it is downright cruel and even fascist, punishing patients with chronic illness and the care providers who step out of 'guidelines' to try out of their humaneness to heal, however improbable the outcome may be.

Physicians who are employed by institutions or abide by medical society guidelines may not, as a result, be allowed to step outside the boundaries of normal care or find the time they need to provide the care they want to provide. They are unable to address the needs of these complex patients and thus, may rationalize their inability or lack of knowledge, and be dismissive and hostile to both the patients and their care providers.

edical policy is not patient-centered, or doctor-centered,

ntered, everyone wins - caregivers can have purpose and

receive care. Financial constraints in academic medical

diminished clinic revenue and increased the pressure

...euze research skills over clinical skills. Thus, enter the tyranny of the randomized controlled trial and the motto, absence of evidence is evidence of absence, until a research gets paid a lot to conduct a big clinical trial - one that owing to its complexity and unpopular topic of chronic infection would never be funded.

The business of research has resulted in grants perpetuating research of one 'fundable' aspect of a disease rather than solving the riddle of disease – real translational medicine. We now have a research infrastructure and funding system paying to do research rather than solving problems or providing care in chronic illness. There are new methods in research design that can enable applied research and these are beginning to catch on.

Yet, out of the ashes of old medical thought and arcane medical specialty societies' power centers a Phoenix rises. It is the rise of the citizen scientist - one who has needs now and wants to get help now. There are now practitioners and researchers who are touched by the needs of this suffering population - the folks who you don't see out at the mall or in the restaurants because they are too sick to be there.

Lyme Savvy is about a psychosocial journey of a patient, my co-author, and a physician, me, on our respective sides of this healing enterprise around a major medical controversy - one in which both sides of the controversy have much to learn about how science progresses.

Some say medical science progresses one funeral at a time - unlike in most fields of science where in modernity innovation is rewarded, in medical science it is first met with hostility. Even our approach to innovation in medical practice is much as Galileo experienced it.

Our goal with *Lyme Savvy* is to help humanize the journey and explain it to others with helpful medical, social, spiritual insights hopefully offering a better framework for healing.

Most importantly, we want to create a dialogue within this controversy with love and compassion for patients who suffer while being healed by care providers who also suffer while providing the healing while policymakers and regulations sit around and figure out how to get their next paycheck.

Dr. B. Robert Mozayeni

February 29, 2016

INTRODUCTION

SHARON

When I started writing this book, my primary goal was to illustrate what my journey with Lyme Disease entailed – from testing to diagnosis to treatment to healing. I wanted to show in detail the complex nature of each step of the lengthy process, breaking down each part so someone reading this could pick up anywhere in the book that corresponds with your place in your healing journey.

When I was first diagnosed I was completely overwhelmed by the information overload. I could not process the data and wasn't sure I even wanted to, as most of what I read was frightening, frustrating and not hopeful.

I needed to be fed the information in bits and pieces. I needed a place to go and look up a word and know I could find out more in one section. The books I found initially were dry and complicated, full of data, whereas I needed to connect emotionally.

I am writing the book I wish I could have read when I was first diagnosed.

While writing this book, I also wanted to provide the latest data and testing information that could help others start their healing journey more quickly and effectively than I did. I was lucky. My uncle Troup told me the laboratories to start with so I could get a head start for my first appointment with Dr. Mozayeni. Being an informed patient can be very empowering. Even as I was finishing this book, I was told of a patient whose physician refused to order any tests from a particular lab because the results were "too difficult to read."

Part of this book focuses more on information and data. But it definitely includes some emotional aspects of my experience, especially in the beginning of my diagnosis. If part of a chapter becomes too dry for you, skip it and move on. There will be a time when you are ready to come back to it. If it's not clicking for you, move ahead and read what interests you. Eventually, it will all make sense and connect for you.

Healing begins with understanding.

I had to understand the disease process. I had to understand chronic illness and the toll it takes on the human body through decades of untreated illness.

I had to understand the importance of finding the cause of the symptoms, not just masking symptoms.

I had to understand what is required to effectively treat this disease.

AUNT BETTY'S STORY

I'm starting this book in the same place of where I started my Lyme journey. The only information I knew about Lyme Disease in 2009 was what I had learned during my Aunt Betty's illness from 2000 until 2002.

My aunt's story is the worst of all stories: refused a lyme test by her internist, she fought for a year to be diagnosed correctly. She had the classic tick bite and EM rash, but because of the arrogance and narrow-mindedness of one physician, Betty could not get the test nor the treatment she needed for a full year.

Before being bitten by a tick in her yard, Betty was a vibrant clinical psychologist and tenured professor, teaching psychology courses to master's level and doctoral candidate students at Auburn University, religiously attending every home football game in her orange and blue. Betty was a "typical" Auburn fan, singing the fight song every week, shouting "War Eagle" when a stronger defense was needed, and crying when the Tigers lost. Betty grew up in Auburn. She earned her undergraduate degree at Auburn. It was home. Teaching at AU was her lifelong dream.

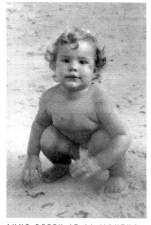

AUNT BETTY AT 11 MONTHS OF AGE

Betty and her husband Troup lived on eight acres on the outskirts of Auburn, Alabama with their horses Sid and Kallie, and their one-eyed goat, Jack. Betty took riding lessons with Kallie on occasion, but mostly, Betty loved nuzzling with her horses and feeding Jack any spare apples she had. She had a good life with a job she loved, a long, happy marriage, a grown son, and a home she and Troup had designed more than a decade earlier. Betty was physically fit, strong, and one of the most attractive women I have ever seen. She could have won any beauty contest with her trim figure, tall stature, and impeccable taste in clothes.

Betty was no wallflower. Her beauty and style brought everyone's eyes to her as she entered any room. She felt throughout her life she didn't necessarily fit in with the crowd, but those around her wanted to fit in with her. She spoke her mind. She would debate and convince those around her to embrace everyone's differences and vulnerabilities.

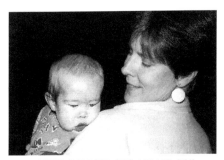

AUNT BETTY HOLDING OUR INFANT SON
STEPHEN (1993)

In June 2000, Betty went to her internist, complaining of a rash starting at her knee. It was 3 inches wide and descended down her calf about 9 inches. He diagnosed it as an allergic reaction to sunscreen. "I know a Paba reaction when I see it," he declared. As to why the rash appeared nowhere else where Betty had applied sunscreen, he had no explanation.

"Do you think it might be Lyme Disease?" Betty asked.

"No, it's not Lyme," he replied. **"We don't have Lyme Disease in Alabama."**

Betty was a strong-willed woman, but she could not convince this physician to order a Lyme test.

Less than two months later, Betty was back in the doctor's office complaining of cramping, twitching, numbness, and her toes drawing up.

Another three months passed. She complained of "both legs not working right" and twitching in her arms, legs, neck, and back. She had foot drop on the left foot, causing her to fall twice. Still, no Lyme test.

Betty tested positive for Lupus, but apparently there was no follow up on this. There is nothing in her medical records or journal about it and Troup didn't recall it being discussed.

Eight months after Betty's initial bull's-eye rash, after a severe decline in her physical health, at Betty's insistence, the internist ran a Lyme test, using the least reliable ELISA test. It was negative. The internist said, "Well, what do you want to do?" Betty asked to see a neurologist.

At a well-known southern teaching university hospital, a neurologist ran a nerve conduction study and diagnosed Betty with ALS. A rash on her leg caused ALS? There is no specific test to diagnose ALS. It is a diagnosis physicians give when they don't know what else to do. It was a death sentence.

Betty and Troup came home devastated. Desperate to better understand ALS and to look for possible alternatives, Troup voraciously researched the Internet and talked with anyone who would talk with him about Betty's symptoms. Remember, this was 2001 when the internet was not quite as filled with information as it is these days. Online research was still laborious and tedious.

This is the point where they learned of IGeneX laboratory in San Diego, California, of their Western blot testing. They went back to the internist and demanded retesting for Lyme from IGeneX. The internist acquiesced and ran the test through IGeneX. Every result came back positive for Lyme. Unfortunately, by this point, Betty's health had declined to the point she was using a walker.

Fourteen months after the initial tick bite, in August 2001, Betty was finally prescribed oral antibiotics for 30 days until a PICC line could be inserted. Her symptoms improved for the first time, though not tremendously.

"She started getting better," Troup later recalls. "It convinced me we were on the right track."

On October 11, 2001 Betty had a PICC line inserted and started i.v. antibiotics. The i.v. Rocephin improved Betty's swallowing and breathing capabilities. In the next phase of treatment, her physician started her on i.v. Azithromycin, which halted the deterioration, but did not improve any of her symptoms. By this point, the infection was too far widespread for any effective advancement.

By March 2002, Betty was in a wheelchair with little feeling in her legs and no strength in her arms. Betty's strength and energy were destroyed. She had gained 50 pounds and was unable to walk. Because of her immobility, she was at high risk for blood clots. She was still taking i.v. antibiotics, which had significantly slowed the progression of her symptoms.

She was still meeting with her doctoral students at her home, consulting with them about their respective theses and internships. She was no longer willing to travel to campus. She was ashamed of her weight gain and wheelchair use. It was the only time her son Terrill had seen the extent of Betty's only character flaw: her vanity. She couldn't bear to be seen in this state.

"Lyme Disease stole my mother's beauty, wisdom, strength, and education," her son Terrill later told me. "It left her with no hope."

On June 5, 2002, Troup was feeding Betty soup for lunch when she simply dropped her head and slumped over. She was dead in an instant with no warning. A blood clot had traveled from her leg to her heart; a pulmonary embolism. There was no way to bring Betty back.

It took a single tick bite less than two years to strip Betty of most physical functions, eventually killing her, and robbing her family, friends, students, and coworkers of her precious talent, heart and laughter.

I share this story **not** to make patients lose hope but rather to validate the experience that I know personally many patients have had. "There is no Lyme Disease in Virginia," a practicing physician stated in 2016, regardless of strong evidence to the contrary. Weekly, I hear stories from frustrated patients about physicians refusing to test for Lyme or stating it is a false positive even though the patient has the tick bite and EM rash.

I share this story to help patients realize sometimes they have to DEMAND to be tested AND to be treated. If you don't get the treatment you need from one physician, find another practitioner who will. Never give up. Keep going until you get the testing and treatment you need to heal.

FROM THERE
TO HERE

Engineering and Medical School

The sciences have always come very naturally to me and I love them. I started reading *Popular Science* in third grade. My grandfather used to take me to the hardware store on weekends and let me buy anything I wanted. I was fascinated with putting things together, learning how they worked. When my mother threw something out because it didn't work anymore, I pulled it from the trash, took it apart, and fixed it. By the time I was eleven, I knew how to run an electrical circuit in the house.

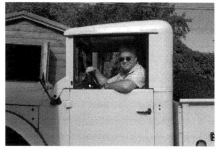

DR. MOZAYENI

I had a lot of physician role models leading me into medicine. My father is a retired surgeon; aunts and uncles in other fields of Medicine. Medicine seemed to be my pathway. I considered engineering for a short while, but I was deeply interested in figuring out how the human machine works.

I attended Union College, a small Liberal Arts college in Upstate New York in conjunction with Albany Medical College that offered an accelerated six-year Bachelor's M.D. program with a liberal arts emphasis.

I was very interested in basic Science from the beginning, particularly research. Biochemistry in med schools involved a lot of memorization and I detested that because they didn't talk about mechanisms. I wanted to know how. I wanted to know why. I didn't want to memorize a set of pathways solely because someone asked me to. I wanted to understand the actual engineering of how these molecules interacted and once I did, then it was very easy for me to remember.

With the liberal arts program, we were required to choose a minor, so I chose Political Science. These courses helped me understand political controversies. I am a scientific student of medical controversies and a political student of scientific controversies. Medicine is full of crazy and intense political controversies. I wanted to understand the science of human nature and politics.

Research and Rheumatology

I am also a research nut. Before I graduated from medical school, I wanted to spend more time in research; I felt like I did not get enough of it in medical school. For almost every year I spent in medical school or medical fellowships or residency, I put in a year working in a basic science research laboratory. During med school, I worked in the Transplant Immunology Lab in the Department of Surgery.

Because I was involved in the Organization of Student

Representatives (OSR) group of the Association of American Colleges (AAMC), I attended a meeting in Chicago of the OSR and AAMC. At that meeting, a representative of the Howard Hughes Medical Institute presented a brand new program called the HHMI-NIH Research Scholars Program.

The Howard Hughes Medical Institute was providing one-to-two year scholarships to medical students who wanted to take a year and work at the National Institutes of Health (NIH) closely with senior NIH scientists. For this, we would earn the equivalent research experience and credentials as an alternative to getting a full Ph.D. The program was called officially the Howard Hughes Medical Institute – National Institutes of Health (HHMI-NIH Research Scholars Program). I applied for its opening year was one of 20 students accepted to it.

After med school I found a research residency program at Yale University. In four years at Yale I did Internal Medicine, one year of a Rheumatology Fellowship and one year of research in the basic Science lab with Professor Frederick Richards of Molecular Biophysics and Biochemistry.

Lyme Disease was discovered by rheumatologists at Yale. Having gone through my whole residency and

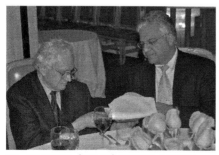

DR. MOZAYENI (RIGHT) HAVING DINNER WITH MARSHALL NIREMBERG, PHD (LEFT). DR. NIREMBERG WON THE NOBEL PRIZE IN MEDICINE FOR DISCOVERY OF THE GENETIC CODE.

fellowship program there, I had not planned on it but I ended up learning a lot about Lyme Disease. At the time there were no major controversies over long-term antibiotic use. We wondered if *Borrelia* responded fully to the antibiotic therapies provided - there was no way to know. And the controversy around long-term antibiotic use had not yet erupted. It was simply a scientific 'given' that there was no way to know if antibiotic therapy had fully treated the infection.

This experience also led me to appreciate inflammatory rheumatic disease can have an infectious basis. In contrast to acute severe infections, chronic infections seemed to bring the patient more often to the attention of the rheumatologist than an infectious disease specialist - remember, **the symptom, not the cause, determines the specialist you see.**

I opened my first practice in 1994 and while I saw some acute Lyme cases here and there and occasionally a chronic Lyme case, it still had not become a major heated controversy. A great physician mentor and colleague of mine, Fred Gill, MD, was then head of our local hospital's "Inflammatory Diseases" section and interviewed me for application to the medical staff. Over the years, he has from time to time advised me on my journey in the management of patients with Lyme Disease.

I founded a biotechnology start up company in 2000 to develop an area of medical science related to the measurement of brain blood flow and develop a big data approach to vascular medicine and human health. I re-entered practice in 2006, knowing I didn't want to go back and do things the managed care way and very much wanted to apply our new medical science about cerebrovascular medicine in clinical practice. I was also interested in learning something new that would help patients with chronic illness – from the perspective of small vessel disease.

I started learning as much as I could about alternative approaches to enhance my awareness of mainstream approaches and the diagnostic science around chronic illness. As a result, I started being identified by the social networks as a #Lyme doc "LLMD" and I started seeing and treating many patients with symptoms consistent with chronic #Lyme, as defined by those social networks.

Coming back into practice was great in many ways but it was also a bit like the astronauts must have felt when they landed on the Planet of the Apes. Everything I thought I knew about Lyme Disease was now a supercharged hostile political controversy with the insurance companies and the Infectious Disease Society of America (IDSA) and insurers using medical boards to stop any physician who was treating patients with Lyme Disease using long-term antibiotics.

It was appalling and it was frightening to suddenly see that what I knew about Lyme Disease had turned into this political nightmare where I literally felt afraid to treat patients for chronic Lyme Disease.

Making the Choice

At some point I had to make a choice. I had to decide whether I wanted to go with a political camp or if I wanted to try to help patients the best way I could. I decided I wanted to help patients. Having been out of practice for a while, I decided the practice wasn't worth coming back to if I couldn't help patients the best way I could and not give up on them.

That's how I see the divide between the doctors who are trying to treat Lyme patients and those who say they don't believe in chronic Lyme Disease. I believe, as a doctor, you make a choice as to whether or not you want to:

A. do everything you can and stick with the patient; or

B. do the consultant thing, you see them for a couple of hours, bill their insurance and tell them you can't help them and then provide them with your strong opinion about how anyone who is trying to help them is a fraud, to slander and libel your colleagues who are actually trying to help the chronically ill patients who have fallen through the cracks and have been failed by the mainstream medical system.

Within a year of coming back into practice and seeing so many Lyme patients, I began to look hard for other explanations for their Lyme Disease. Based on my previous research and experience with patients with small-vessel disease, I knew they had small vessel disease. I had observations clinically from a good neuro exam -

hard data that I could see for myself. It kept me searching for a better answer to explain the controversy.

As a result of that searching, I uncovered the presence of *Bartonella* and some other co-infections. I believe their presence contributes to the symptoms and signs of small-vessel disease and that they may indeed be the missing piece of the puzzle.

With the conviction of my own physical exam I knew I was looking for signs causing small-vessel disease. I was not of the mindset that these patients had psychiatric causes because I understood small-vessel disease enough to know one of the first manifestations of small vessel disease is mild cognitive impairment caused by subcortical disconnection caused by small-vessel disease limiting blood flow to the interconnecting neurons of the brain in the deeper white matter tracts and neuro-inflammation. And we know inflammation deplete neurotransmitters and nitro-oxide by depleting biopterin.

When they get some mild cognitive impairment, these patients get very anxious. Their adrenaline levels surge. They develop adrenal fatigue, and generally insomnia and severe fatigue. One thing leads to another, leads to another, leads to another and before you know it you've got multisystem disease.

One of the biggest problems in any antibiotic trial in Lyme Disease is if you give only antibiotics to these people who have multisystem involvement, they don't get better. In fact,

patients often get worse until you manage them from a comprehensive view involving principles of integrative medicine, functional medicine, and mainstream medicine and very good new emerging tools in diagnostic medical science.

I knew these patients had psychiatric disease as a result of their small-vessel disease; it wasn't that they had a personality disorder. It was not "all in their head" but "*also* in their head."

In 2007, a patient of mine was asked by his internist to see an Infectious Disease specialist. This particular well-known ID specialist told my patient Lyme Disease was a psychiatric disease, a personality disorder. This non-psychiatrist determined that chronic Lyme was a psychiatric disease. This comment infuriated me then and it infuriates me even today. I knew it was a small-vessel disease based on my exam, background and history in vascular inflammatory diseases, and research that produced patents and peer-reviewed publications on cerebrovascular disease.

A Fortunate Meeting

As I started looking for better tools to look at the various co-infections associated with Lyme, I realized that while we had some testing for *Borrelia* and for *Babesia*, we had hardly any good test for *Bartonella*. Following my instincts in medical research and science, I started trying to hunt down better *Bartonella* tests.

A veterinarian I worked with who had been active in Lyme Disease, Dr. Wendy Walker, was also on this quest to look for a better *Bartonella* test. Dr. Walker and another patient of mine introduced me to professor Ed Breitschwerdt, DVM. The very first phone call we had ended up lasting to two hours. It started off by my explaining my situation to Ed. He said the more he studied *Bartonella* the less he felt he knew. That is when I knew I had found the right research collaborator.

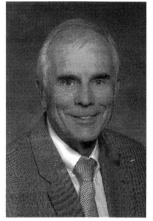

DR. ED BREITSCHWERDT, DVM

Ed suggested, "Why don't you start sending a few specimens and we will run some tests for those patients?" I had numerous patients I wanted to send for testing. So I figured I would send them until he told me to stop. I sent maybe a hundred before he called me one day.

That Research Discovery Moment

He said, "In veterinarians who we think are at high risk for *Bartonella*, we find a high prevalence, but in your patients we are seeing a rate of *Bartonella* that is considerably higher, almost double what we are seeing in veterinarians. There is something about your patient group that seems to place them at a much higher risk for *Bartonella* than our veterinarians."

That is when he and I both had the *aha! moment* about the possibility chronic Lyme was actually being greatly contributed to or even caused substantially by *Bartonella*. We still don't have a clear sense on how much of it is *Borrelia* versus *Bartonella* versus *Protozoa*.

But the more I study chronic Lyme the more I think *Bartonella* is a significant and important public health problem.

Recent data from the CDC showed even they had underestimated its prevalence.

That project with Ed ended up with our publishing the results of *Bartonella* testing in 296 patients who felt they could have had chronic Lyme Disease as defined by their social networks. Some of them had arthritic symptoms. Some of them had rheumatoid arthritis. Most had Central Nervous System evidence of small vessel disease. What we found is described in the paper we published in the CDC's journal, *Emerging Infectious Disease* in May of 2012. The Lyme group at the CDC was disturbed by our paper attempting to clarify the problem and tried to discredit it in a letter to the editor. We appreciated the chance to rebut their letter.

I started trying to treat these patients looking at the best available treatment protocols and *in vitro* sensitivity studies, being guided by very little good science around how to best treat *Bartonella* because we have never really had a good way to detect it in the first place. I struggled to find the best treatment protocol. After treating patients who were positive for *Bartonella* I found we had a fairly high success rate. To date, out of a few hundred patients I have only had a small number of confirmed laboratory-documented cases of recurrence of *Bartonella* after my treatment protocol.

From a medical science and discovery point of view, we know there have been cases of *Bartonella* published over the years but no physician has published an extensive case series. Thanks to the research collaboration with Dr. Breitschwerdt and his team, the largest case series worldwide in *Bartonella* has been published. It all came from applying what I knew about medical science to finding the best possible new treatment pathways for patients who had a desperate need for solutions.

I never planned to become an expert clinician regarding *Bartonella* – it happened because of the combination of;

1. the analytical thinking as a physician–scientist, and

2. being compassionate and maintaining the courage to be compassionate in a hostile medical climate.

Seeing the Whole Patient

My style of learning and understanding the physics, physical chemistry and physiology of how the body works is a visual-spatial approach. I have a visual-spatial capability to see what's happening. When I interview a patient I am literally building in my mind a holographic model of what the patient

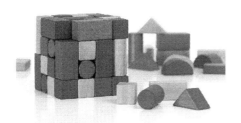

has and the situation they are in. I think about how if I change one thing on one side of the hologram, what would happen on the other side. In my mind I naturally, intuitively 'see' the interconnections of the different aspects of an individual's health.

My definition of compassion is to hold the thought and potential outcome for a patient until they can do so themselves.

I try to envision their ideal state, what the hologram would ideally look like, understand what their state is presently, and then try to move them from the state of illness. I view it as growth from a condition the patient is not happy with and wants to evolve out of and improve. Many patients are not necessarily in a situation where they are ready to move out of the phase, for one reason or another. With every patient, I try to understand what goes into the situation they are in, feeling what they are feeling and whatever else goes into that equation.

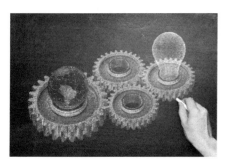

What I have is a systems view; the kind of overview approach taken by engineers. I need to understand all the parts, how the parts relate to the overall and to one another. Only with that view in mind can I proceed to figure out and prioritize the treatment recommendations. As I move a patient from one 'state' to another I must understand what needs to happen first. This is the hardest part requiring knowledge, skill, and experience.

Emotional and spiritual components must be included in the entire hologram of the system's view of the patient's illness. This is because:

> **You cannot heal chronic illness unless you address the body, the mind and the soul.**

I could have done a short three-to-five year residency and gone right into standard-of-care medical practice, followed guidelines and only what the algorithms told me that I could help. If I had done that, then we wouldn't have put *Bartonella* on the map and understood it is a medically significant infection for humans.

The Path to Dr. Mozayeni

When I was originally diagnosed with Lyme Disease, someone told me about a neighbor who also had it. I knew this person. I called her up and asked her for help. She seemed empathic during our conversation, but I found it strange she was unwilling to give me her physician's name and number. And she didn't seem interested in "helping" me in any way other than to say, "I'm sorry you have this horrible disease."

When I hung up the phone, I felt lost and even more alone. I promised myself I would never do that to another person. Then I got a phone call from a good friend.

"You have got to talk to my boss!" she declared. "He has Lyme Disease too and he has this amazing physician." I met her boss, Dan. We talked over coffee a couple of times. He told me his long winding story to a *Bartonella* diagnosis and his healing experience with Dr. Mozayeni, I was convinced. I made my appointment and never once regretted my decision.

Dan and I now meet for coffee every six weeks or so to catch up on one another. He remains a good friend and a great source of support. Now, I try to offer the same to anyone who calls or emails me.

I know what it is like to be newly diagnosed and have nowhere to turn. I know what it is like not to understand the #Lyme "jargon." I know what it is like to wonder what treatment protocols are offered and how to tell them apart. I get it. Having this disease is often emotionally isolating and physically painful. I can't reduce people's pain levels, but I can let them know they are not alone.

You are not alone.
You are not crazy.
You have a legitimate illness.
You can heal from this disease.

It took eight years of migrating, mysterious symptoms before I knew to ask for a Lyme test in the summer of 2009. After another misdiagnosis (Lupus), my uncle called me, "You don't have Lupus. You have Lyme Disease. You need to get a Western blot blood test from IGeneX laboratory."

Lyme Disease? Don't you get that from a tick?

My aunt died from Lyme Disease. I watched Aunt Betty fight just to get tested; and then to get treated. I suddenly realized even though this infection had killed someone close to me, I didn't know anything about it.

Lyme Disease? Really?

I never go outside. I hate getting sweaty; I hate getting dirty. I get sunburned too easily. I don't have any outdoor hobbies. How could I get a tick bite? How could I possibly have Lyme Disease?

Uncle Troup called me multiple times over the next few weeks, slowly, meticulously educating me on the disease, the diagnosis process, and finding the right physician (a Lyme Literate Medical Doctor or LLMD for short). The urgency in his voice was palpable.

"Why do I have to get the Lyme test at IGeneX?" I asked.

"It's the only lab in the United States with a reliable test," Troup replied. "When you use any other lab, their results can be up to 60 percent inaccurate with false negatives."

"So why does everyone use the other labs?" I asked. "Why waste the money?"

"Insurance," Troup answered. I heard this one word response more than once over the next few months when asking why.

"Don't waste your time with any doctor but an LLMD," he sternly warned. I heard the warning, but I couldn't find an LLMD who could see me quickly. I had to wait a month. I made the appointment, but in the meantime, I saw a rheumatologist. She listened to my history, did a physical exam.

"No swelling in the joints," she noted.

"No, but they are tender and painful," I replied. "I can't walk up or down the stairs anymore."

"You are still very flexible. You have good range of motion," she observed out loud.

"Yes, but I am much less flexible than I used to be. In the morning, it takes me 20 minutes of stretching just to be able to get out of bed," I explained.

She drew blood, but it was not sent to IGeneX. Two bands tested positive for Lyme.

"No Lyme," she said. She didn't know what I had, but whatever it was, she couldn't help me. She stated, "no need for a follow up appointment."

I heard about another rheumatologist who was supposedly good with autoimmune issues. I gave him my thick file, which he refused to open. He listened to five minutes of my history, interrupted me, and declared I had bursitis in my hip. He gave me a shot of cortisone in my hip and told me to come back in three weeks for another shot. My hip actually felt better after the shot, but three weeks later, the pain returned threefold worse.

An osteopath looked through my thick file and listened to my story. He drew my blood and sent it to IGeneX. It came back with five bands positive for Lyme. A week after the results arrived, he called me. But in our seven-minute phone conversation on a Friday afternoon, he emphatically denied Lyme.

"What do we do from here then?" I asked.

"We treat you symptomatically and hope the peripheral neuropathy doesn't worsen."

"But what if it does worsen like it has over the past few months?" I queried.

"I guess if it does, we'll run more tests," he replied. I brought him back to the Lyme.

"Is it possible to have a co-infection of Lyme?"

"Well, yes, it's possible. But it's so rare, I don't test for co-infections." That is exactly what Aunt Betty's internist said about Lyme.

Good-bye.

If it had not been for Uncle Troup's insistence I would not have pressed beyond that last phone call. I am not sure I would have kept the appointment with the LLMD. But I did keep the appointment. I owe Troup my life.

Meeting with Dr. Mozayeni is unlike any conversation I have ever had with other physicians. It was a new beginning for me; the start of one of the most empowering experiences of my life. Later in this book, I will discuss more in depth the details of our first appointment.

Dr. Mozayeni's treatment protocol is healing my body. His compassion and dry humor are healing my soul. He is giving me my life back, and my family's life back, as my husband, son and three other family members also have co-infections of Lyme Disease.

Finding the Right Diagnosis and the Right Treatment

I hope this book helps others find the right diagnosis, and even more importantly, the right treatment.

I hope practitioners will read this book and become more knowledgeable and aggressive in considering Lyme Disease, co-infections, or small vessel disease as a possible diagnosis. I hope they will test for Lyme Disease **and** co-infections using only the most recent reliable laboratories.

I pray no one else will suffer as many others have and do; nor die. I hope by telling Aunt Betty's story and my story, patients will see the breadth of conditions that can all be symptoms of small vessel disease.

I believe readers will each take away what they need from this book. Every healing experience is different. What works for me does not always work for my husband or son. What works for my nieces does not necessarily work for me. Oddly enough, what works for me now may not have worked a year ago. And vice versa.

This field of medicine is dynamic, evolving, discovering new infections and parasites and developing treatment protocols for each.

To fully heal, I must remain willing to participate in all possible solutions rather than wallow in the frustration of the disease process.

What did not work a year ago might work now with a new combination or dosage.

If any of my story or Aunt Betty's story sounds like a portion of yours, I strongly encourage you to get tested by one of the nation's leading laboratories. Get a copy of your results, and then find a good Lyme Literate Medical Doctor (LLMD).

There IS hope.
There IS healing.

WHAT DO WE ALL WANT?

To Be Able to Grocery Shop

SHARON

Of all the things affecting a patient's perspective on their quality of life, going to the grocery store is most often listed as the number one item. If a patient cannot get to the grocery store and shop for food, self-care becomes limited. Not everyone has someone else who can run the errands. And even those who do, the mere fact that running

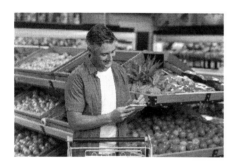

in to get a few items is not an option results in a constricting lifestyle. And, if a patient is already cognitively impaired, forgetful, then trying to remember the grocery list whether for him/herself or someone else becomes an even more critical issue.

This one task, grocery shopping, illuminates how basic life becomes for a chronically ill patient.

Most patients reading this book are probably asking one or more of the following:

"How can I heal from this disease?"

"*Can* I heal from this disease?"

"What disease do I have?"

"How long will it take me to heal?"

"Will I ever feel normal again?"

"*How* do I heal from this disease?"

When I started into treatment, I wanted to find out what was causing my pain and get rid of that pain. I wanted to feel better. I wanted to heal. I wanted to trust a physician.

As treatment has progressed I want more. I want my family to heal. I want my friends and extended family to understand the disease I have and to respect the seriousness of the damage it can inflict. I want to educate everyone on how rampant the spread of small vessel disease is. I want my fellow Lyme patients' suffering to end or at least subside. I want everyone to experience the healing I am having.

Every healing experience is different.

Do not give up.

And aim for nothing less than a complete cure.

Essential Players

The essential players in the relationship that is the essence of the doctor-patient relationship in this chronic disease model are:

- the patient,
- the practitioner,
- the patient's family and friends,

- the practitioner's office staff and
- the practitioner's family and friends.

There are layers beyond this, such as other practitioners the patient is seeing and the patient's community. The good health of the individual improves the health of the community and prevents bad things from happening in that community. A healed person positively impacts someone else and you get an effect two-to-three layers past the individual close in the circle.

Putting Yourself First

You may be the primary caregiver in your family. If you are, you first need to make sure you are in good shape. If you don't, then no one is taken care of.

Many of our patients are moms. They have responsibilities, kids, etc. They often exhibit their illness at a time of the greatest stress in their life during the time frame when they have young families.

A caregiver has, above all other things, to learn to love themselves and to be kind to themselves and to nurture themselves. It is hard for a few reasons.
- They are not used to doing so, because they have dependents.
- They don't have time to do it.
- If they knew how to do it, they forgot.
- They always think something or someone else is more important.

Caregivers tend never to be highest on their own priority list even though it is completely logical for individual caregivers to focus on taking care of themselves first. They may also think they cannot appear too happy if someone else is not happy. They do not realize if they were happy, the other person would actually feel relieved because they have someone taking care of them who is centered.

When someone has a caregiver, it is also important the caregiver be emotionally and energetically centered. They are likely to have integrity when it comes to their thoughts, their work and their process. They are positive and healthy.

It is important then to be respectful and supportive of our caregivers, whether it is our mother or some health care worker who is doing all they can to help you. When it comes to taking care of our patients, we want to foster centeredness; and we would like to see it in all of the parties involved in the patient's care.

I find the patients who are the most successful at getting better are those who are helped by the medical team to be more centered; to have their needs met.

Fulfillment, Feeling Centered

At the end of the day, what do we all want? We want to feel fulfilled – that we matter.

If you are a patient, you want to heal and feel well. You want to be able to go back to doing the things you want to do. You want to be able to take care of the people you want to take care of. You want to be able to do things to show your love for the people you love, for your family, for your friends.

As a practitioner you want to feel fulfilled. You want to know you made a difference. You want to receive feedback that you made a difference.

We want patients <u>and</u> practitioners to feel more centered. We want the professionals to feel fulfilled and to have a livelihood so they want to come back and do an even better job the next day.

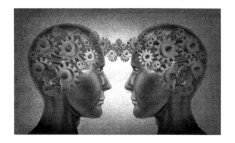

It is a shared responsibility between the patient and the practitioner. Each has to do their part and they have to do it every day in an effective collaborative way. All involved have to be communicative; they have to be respectful of others, of their time, their resources, and their limitations. I think if one does so, you develop some really wonderful and satisfying relationships.

WHAT'S THE SECRET TO HEALING?

SHARON

When I started on this part of my healing journey in 2009, I kept asking people what treatments they were doing, what meds they were taking, what detoxes they did, etc. I wanted to know THE SECRET. I wanted to know HOW TO HEAL. There *had* to be a secret recipe, a secret combination. If I knew what it was, I could do it, take it, use it... and heal.

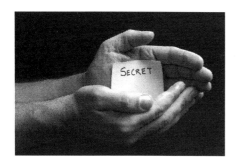

I have since learned a few things I want to share here. Because now, I am the one being asked, "What protocol are you using?", "What detoxes worked best for you?", "What alternative therapies were successful for you?" While I am happy to answer the questions, I know the answers are not simple.

The same treatments and medications
do not necessarily work for everyone.
There is no one answer.
There is no one cure.
There is no one protocol.
It is different for every single patient out there.

That sucks, doesn't it? I know. I agree. I WISH I could give you the secret recipe right here. I wish I could tell you which meds to take, which supplements to use, how long to use each, which detox to do, which alternative therapies to try.

I will tell you what I have seen as successful trends or commonalities in those who are healing.

Please note I know some people who have healed from chronic illness who do NOT fit into these characteristics. There are exceptions to every "rule." The following is merely a generalization from what I have witnessed in myself and in others during these past years.

I believe the following elements of the healing process are critical:

Diagnosis

Diagnosis is usually made by a well-trained Lyme Literate Medical Doctor who understands the comprehensive nature of the infection and co-infections, and systemic affects, and places the person above the guidelines.

The patient is tested for co-infections using the best labs in the nation with the latest, most modern technologies available (i.e., Galaxy Diagnostics, Fry Labs, IGeneX).

The patient is interviewed thoroughly and examined for clinical symptoms.

Physician Criteria

The physician is well trained in the treatment of Lyme Disease.

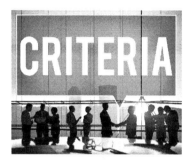

The physician should be current on latest research and incorporate changes to treatment protocols when necessary. What was used four years ago or even one year ago might not be what should be used today.

The physician's treatment protocols align more closely to ILADS rather than IDSA. Physicians and patients in surveys have indicated their preference for ILADS guidelines.

The physician invites and expects the patient to participate actively in the treatment protocol as a team member.

The physician is compassionate, kind, and non-judgmental (and usually has a good sense of humor).

The physician is willing to say "I don't know," and then work toward an analytical solution.

Patient Personality Traits

- The patient is 100 percent determined to reach a cure and will not let anything stand in their way.

- The patient does not drink alcohol or abuse drugs to self-medicate.

- The patient does not smoke.

- The patient limits sugar intake.

- The patient continues to set goals despite feeling less than perfect.

- The patient is willing to try new things, willing to trust the physician, willing to go to any lengths to heal.

- The patient is 100 percent honest and forthright with the physician.

- The patient is compliant with treatment.

- The patient puts his/her physical, mental/emotional, and spiritual well being above all else.

- The patient asks for help when it is needed; *and accepts the help when it is offered.*

- The patient keeps a positive attitude.

- The patient never gives up.

Antibiotic Treatment

The patient is treated with long-term oral antibiotics and/or anti-parasitic medications specific to the types of infections and *Protozoa* for which they have tested positive.

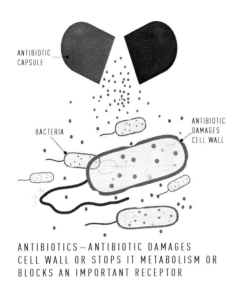

ANTIBIOTICS—ANTIBIOTIC DAMAGES CELL WALL OR STOPS IT METABOLISM OR BLOCKS AN IMPORTANT RECEPTOR

The antibiotics are titrated up gradually. If multiple antibiotics are prescribed, they are not started all at once and not initially at full dosage.

Ancillary Physical Therapies

The patient incorporates some type(s) of physical therapies to remind the body of what it can do, to prepare it for the healing process.

Psychological Therapies

The patient incorporates psychological therapies, creating solutions to previously unresolved psychological issues.

Alternative Therapies

The patient utilizes some alternative therapies, which may, for them, reduce the severity of symptoms, shorten the healing process, open pathways into new ways of healing.

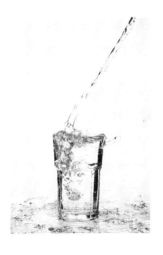

Dietary Changes

The patient maintains a diet of almost all organic foods, focused more upon an alkaline, vegetable based diet; also decreasing or completely eliminating intake of sugar, soy, gluten, and dairy products.

Community

The patient surrounds him/herself with people who are positive, supportive, kind, and compassionate; all attributes are helpful to healing.

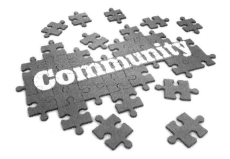

The patient laughs every day; really laughs.

The patient encourages others on their own pathways to healing.

Spiritual

The patient finds a positive, spiritual connection to a power greater than him/herself.

The patient finds a way to live life based on healing, love, compassion, and health.

The patient finds forgiveness for all transgressions and offers forgiveness to all transgressors.

The patient reaches out and finds a way to heal spiritually and emotionally, careful not to participate in victimizing behavior.

Family Warning

This is probably the most blunt section in this book. If your spouse, significant other, parents, or whomever is closest to you is not involved in your care, is not asking to speak to your physician, is not going to any appointments with you, is not supporting you at home in your efforts to heal, you should seek counseling immediately.

For too many years, I have witnessed too many patients whose family members have impeded and hurt their care. Too many patients have seen relentless cruelty from the spouse. Too many patients have been the brunt of long, expensive, deceitful, divorces often perpetuated by divorce lawyers who delight in billing for as many hours as possible.

I have witnessed too many patients who have been attacked in every way possible, often involving any children the couple may have. I have witnessed too many patients' time, financial and emotional resources depleted.

The death of this already unhealthy relationship can become the most significant and worst impediment to healing. But until that unhealthy relationship is dissolved, true healing cannot occur. This may be one of those things that is inevitable and necessary for long term healing but it can also blindside many patients.

Let me reiterate here that the above list of items is *not* what helps everyone. This is merely a list of commonalities I have noticed among most of those who are healing. There are always exceptions and variations.

SEPARATING LYME DISEASE & *BARTONELLA*

❝I have an almost complete disregard of precedent and a faith in the possibility of something better. It irritates me to be told how things always have been done. I defy the tyranny of precedent. I cannot afford the luxury of a closed mind. I go for anything new that might improve the past.❞

– CLARA BARTON

HISTORY OF
LYME DISEASE

Discovery of Lyme Disease

A pediatrician in Old Lyme, Connecticut, was noticing a particular form of arthritis in the children. Epidemiological teams were brought in, one team led by Dr. Allen Steere and others in the Rheumatology Department at Yale, looking at the community, the kids, and the environment. They looked, characterized and then named it Lyme Disease after the town. Secondarily, through the work of the Connecticut State Health Department, other epidemiologists and Dr. Willy Burgdorfer, the microbe was identified and named *Borrelia burgdorferi*, after Dr. Burgdorfer.

Antibody Testing Developed

That discovery led to some diagnostic tests based on the presence of antibodies in the blood directed against parts of the bacterium. When you look at different antibodies in the blood one test is done using a method, called the Western blot, or sometimes a protein immunoblot.

The classic medical definition of Lyme Disease is that condition which results from *Borrelia burgdorferi,* the bacterium being inoculated into the skin by the deer tick, *Ixodes dammini.*

How Lyme is Transferred to the Human Body

The deer tick carries *Borrelia burgdorferi* (and other microbes) in its gut and its saliva. After it bites, as it becomes more and more engorged, it is more likely to reflux the blood back into the body. Therefore the risk of exposure or inoculation with the microbe increases exponentially with the amount of time the tick is attached, as it becomes engaged.

Initially the blood moves into the tick. Later, as the tick becomes engorged, the blood can move both ways and therefore the risk of contracting *Borrelia* increases exponentially with attachment duration. This has led many to the belief that if the tick is only attached very briefly, it is relatively unlikely to transmit Lyme Disease, which in turn has led to some falsely held dogma among physicians — that because it is *less likely* it is *impossible*. It is not only theoretically possible that brief attachment can transmit *Borrelia,* but there have been some clinical examples of this, as well.

When there is an exposure, the risk of transmittal is a probability between 0 and 100%. It is not a certainty; it is not a certainty at 48 hours nor is it a certainty that it does not happen at one hour. It is simply more likely over time to transmit the *Borrelia burgdorfi* bacteria and other microbes.

When it does happen, we currently believe the *Borrelia* then gets into the skin and spreads in a radial pattern outward from the tick bite. Redness is most intense at the leading front of the microbe spreading outward through the skin. The little band that is a little bit more red than the surrounding area is the band that makes the whole thing look like a bull's-eye or a target lesion.

There are not multiple rings within the ring, like a real bulls-eye. There is simply a bite with redness and then there is a faint ring around it. Sometimes the ring is very intense. This rash is typically called a bull's-eye rash or the scientific term, erythema chronicum migrans (ECM), which literally means redness slowly moving. Just because it has a Latin term does not necessarily convey any extra wisdom or deep understanding about the microbe or disease process. The name is purely descriptive.

DIAGNOSIS OF
LYME DISEASE

DR. MOZAYENI

Clinical Diagnosis of Lyme

In my medical view the word Lyme represents a Connecticut town and a rash that may be associated with joint pain and/or neurological symptoms. Clinically, the only way you can be certain you are dealing with Lyme Disease is:

- *if you have the history story of the right kind of tick exposure,*
- *the erythema chronicum migrans creates a bull's-eye lesion and, of course,*
- *if a person also gets sick from it and develops arthritis.*

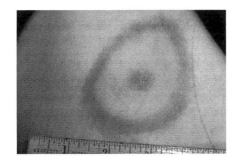

When you have these elements in the development of the illness, there is no lab test that can be better than this history to help you with the diagnosis. If the clinical story is there, there really is no point in relying on a lab test to prove it or to disprove it. But better tests help physicians and patients become more comfortable with the diagnosis – or more confused!

I have seen many cases where a negative test was used to claim there was no Lyme Disease. Clinically, the only time we can really be certain we are dealing with Lyme Disease is when the events I just described happen in that sequence with that rash.

This simple truth was ignored often enough by doctors that the Commonwealth of Virginia had to pass a law telling doctors how they must interpret a negative test for Lyme. It is sad some doctors need laws to remind them of very basic concepts in medical science, such as test sensitivity, specificity, and predictive value.

Blood Test for Lyme

At the time of the tick bite and the rash, if someone has never been exposed to *Borrelia* before, they will not have antibodies to the *Borrelia* microbe. It takes usually six to twelve weeks to see antibodies to *Borrelia.* These antibodies initially develop as IgM, within two to four weeks and then later as IgG within six to 12 weeks or more. For Bartonella, it can be months and may never happen or decrease over time in the majority of patients (Maggi RG, Mozayeni BR, Pultorak EL, et al. **Bartonella Spp. Bacteremia And Rheumatic Symptoms In Patients From Lyme Disease-Endemic Region**. *Emerging Infectious Diseases.* May 2012; 18(5):783 791. http://www.ncbi.nlm.nih.gov/pmc/articles/PMC3358077/).

To evaluate a tick bite, the first test we do is the Western blot. It should first be done within a week or two of the exposure, **before** the exposure causes antibodies. This is to determine what the **baseline** antibody level was before the bite. **It does not yet reflect antibodies produced as a result of the *Borrelia* exposure.**

Typically, 2-3 months later one would re-test for *Borrelia* by the Western blot to see if there has been a **change** in the antibody response between the initial and the 12-week post-bite test.

Bayesian Probability Decision Making

I want to make an important point here: Many clinicians and patients don't understand it takes time (weeks) to produce antibodies. I have seen many errors of diagnosis being made when the clinical history was classic for Lyme Disease and strongly diagnostic. When you have a high probability of Lyme Disease before any testing, that probability cannot be altered by the result of a negative test because the prior probability was so high. This is called 'predictive value' and it is a form of Bayesian probability decision-making. It is the standard clinicians should use to make decisions.

Lately, Bayesian adaptive clinical trials have become the leading edge method for conducting clinical research. It is all about probabilities. You have to know what your prior probability was before an event occurs in order to gauge whether or not that event really matters in your updated probability estimate after a test outcome is observed.

In the case of a clear-cut tick exposure, ECM rash and *Borrelia*, you can be certain you have Lyme and a negative test result should not change your mind.

The world of diagnostic testing is really a world of probabilities and probabilities in context. When you introduce a bias as to whether or not someone has post-Lyme syndrome or persistent Lyme, you are already prejudicing your test results because you are already changing your prior determination using a method that was not optimized to rule out Lyme Disease.

In numerous consultations, I encountered physicians who had told their patient (who had a clear-cut positive Western blot test for Lyme) that because their clinical history didn't match, they couldn't possibly have Lyme Disease. I have also seen them look at a strongly positive result and say it can't be right, it's false, all because the clinician could not or didn't want to deal with the problem.

I have also seen physicians look at a clearly negative result and tell the patient, "No, it can't be right because your risk is high."

Sometimes the judgment is right; sometimes it is off base because of biases in regard to whether or not the patient's symptoms are believed to really exist.

If a doctor believes everyone who has been treated has post-Lyme syndrome with no persistent microbe and that no other microbe other than *Borrelia* co-infection has been missed, then their bias is to take any positive result no matter how strong it is and say it is false. I have seen it happen. In other words, they 'see it when they believe it.'

There are some very important and new emerging diagnostic tests beginning to shed light on how some of the symptoms a patient has may be from other infections than *Borrelia* even though they may clearly have *Borrelia*. We will discuss these tests later in the book.

Considering Other Ailments

When you look at a patient who has post-Lyme syndrome or chronic Lyme Disease, you have to challenge yourself to make sure you identify every process that could be causing the patient's condition. If it is infections, you need to broaden your scope and not be single-mindedly with tunnel vision looking at *Borrelia*. A few possible causes include food allergies, hypothyroidism, adrenal fatigue, and MTHFR Genetic Traits (These will be covered in more detail elsewhere in this book.).

In general, when a doctor treats a lot of patients for Lyme Disease, everything starts looking like a nail for his hammer. Patients have to look for physicians treating Lyme Disease who don't have a bias against it but who are also very thorough about trying to uncover any other possible explanation for the symptoms the patient is experiencing.

Often, even with evidence of infection, a physician must consider other possible explanations for the symptoms, especially when these other diagnoses are usually easier to treat.

LYME TREATMENT BASICS

Traditional Tick Bite Treatment

The diagnosis of Lyme Disease is not simple and neither is treatment.

Let's move out three months from the original tick bite and classic ECM rash. Now we have a patient who is ill and the antibody tests are still not clearly positive. In the meanwhile, that person has already had the standard short protocol of doxycycline because a practitioner wanted to allay the patient's concerns even though the Western blot done in the beginning was negative as expected (before antibodies develop).

Let's assume the Western blot has slightly changed, but not in any way that convinces anyone. In other words, they might have one new IgG band or maybe the total antibody, or the EIA, is now slightly positive or weakly positive.

Now we have this symptom complex, and it is not clear. In other words, there is no other explanation and we cannot prove it is from the original event. At this point, doctors who believe that only a two-week protocol is necessary start calling this post-Lyme syndrome. They may not call it that until it is a few more months out. They might give the person up to 30 days of doxycycline. They might even add another antibiotic if that didn't work. But to those who believe antibiotics are uniformly 100% effective against *Borrelia* there is no other explanation other than calling symptoms the patients experience 'post-Lyme syndrome.'

Other physicians are apt to believe it is common sense that this patient still has Lyme Disease because the patient originally had the tick bite with the diagnostic ECM rash. At this point, because there is no other explanation, we need to simply intensify or extend the treatment for chronic Borreliosis. The alternative is to abandon the patient with nothing to offer.

The point to make about this debate is it can exist only in the absence of good information. You can easily have an argument over what it is and what it isn't because you really don't have any way to disprove or prove either theory. So people argue over whose evidence is bigger and better.

If a practitioner is also consulting Infectious Disease specialists you feel like you are starting to go out on a limb and potentially risk professional sanctions if this patient has an adverse reaction to the medications. If you are a patient, you are terrified that your doctor is worried more about his professional sanctions than about giving you the proper treatment.

If, as the practitioner, you always try to do the best you can for the patient, then your good intentions **should** carry the day. But you may still be persecuted by medical 'peers' and medical boards even if the patient gets better; sad, but true.

Patient Preference

From the patient's point of view, additional and more intense treatment is the way to go. If you subject this to a rigorous evidence-based medicine (EBM) analysis, according to Canadian medical doctor and pioneer David L. Sackett, you must acknowledge patient preference is a very important determinant of the evidence database,

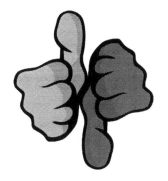

because **the perception of benefit and harm is the patient's**.

Rarely do medical policy makers consider patient preference in evidence-based medicine guidelines.

Gauging the Value of a Treatment

When you are gauging the value of a treatment, there are two measures. One is called the number needed to harm (NNH). In other words how many patients do you have to treat before you harm someone? The other one is the number needed to treat (NNT) to see benefit. The NNT is how many do you have to treat in order to help someone? The numbers are out of 100. For example, out of 100 people you would treat with a longer course of antibiotic, what fraction will have a significant adverse reaction and how do you compare that to the number who will have a significant positive reaction?

The number of patients needed to treat and the number needed to harm are the way we measure the efficacy and risk of any treatment. But the perception of what constitutes benefit and harm belongs to the patient with guidance and information from the physician. This point is extremely critical and central to evidence-based medicine, but it is completely lost on the medical professionals and policy makers who would rather weigh in with a top-down dogmatic and paternalistic view of how things should be done. In a free society this should not be unless the public is clearly and immediately harmed.

We are now at the point of dealing with this patient who either has post-Lyme syndrome or chronic Lyme Disease depending on whether or not you choose to look at it from the patient's or the doctor's point of view. This is because the patient will prefer, usually, to take a chance to have full recovery over a death or disability sentence.

EMERGING AWARENESS: IT'S NOT ALWAYS JUST LYME *(BORRELIA)*

Differing Perspectives and Priorities

Now we are in a situation where we have different perspectives and different priorities competing between the medical establishment view and the patient-centric view of the evidence base around this entire problem. How do we move on from here, not only for an individual patient but for this entire controversy in general? There are different layers to this question.

One layer is simply that with better diagnostic testing we have more clarity on what is actually going on with these patients. We have more accurate information and can make the right decisions. In that category, we have the hope and promise of continued better diagnostic testing for *Borrelia, Bartonella* and various other 'co-infections' in the vector microbiome.

Another layer of this to recognize: that to complete a full evidence-based medicine analysis, you must rigorously incorporate patient preference in your evidence if you are to be considered a valid authority in Lyme Disease in a free society.

If you do a more formal evidence-based analysis, you also include the evidence that you gain by talking to expert clinicians who treat these conditions. You cannot simply cite the lack of randomized control trials. You have to consider patient preference and you have to consider current, contemporary expert experience.

The third layer is to understand the biology; in this case, small-vessel disease often is in fact created by chronic infections other than *Borrelia*, such as *Bartonella*, and this co-infection can cause many neurovascular symptoms.

SHARON

When I initially tested positive for Lyme, I was confused by the fact I hardly spent anytime outside, I didn't recall ever being bitten by a tick and had never seen a bull's eye rash on my skin. I thought in order to have Lyme Disease, I had to have all three of the above.

My first appointment with Dr. Mozayeni was my introduction into co-infections and small vessel disease. No, I didn't understand it all in the first appointment. But I understood enough for it to make sense for almost every symptom I had experienced during the thirty years prior.

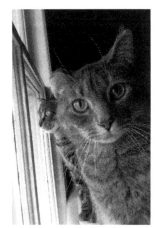

Cats are *Bartonella's* primary carrier. I owned cats my entire life; I knew it was more likely for me to have *Bartonella* than Lyme Disease. I listened intently when Dr. Mozayeni explained his research and what

©JENNIFER TINNES

he had discovered thus far. It was like a giant jigsaw puzzle suddenly fitting together into a beautiful, clear picture. Every piece melded together. Every symptom qualified for the diagnosis of *Bartonella*.

Now we needed the blood work to show it.

DR. MOZAYENI

This is where we must distinguish between Lyme Disease and the social networking term #Lyme Disease. These are two very different definitions that must be reconciled.

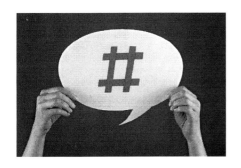

When patients have concerns about Lyme, they think about #Lyme Disease in the broadest sense of having many symptoms but with a narrow focus on *Borrelia* itself. While other infections may be considered they are always just called co-infections; the emphasis is usually placed on the *Borrelia* rather than all the other possibilities. **The possibility that the co-infection may be the main infection** is not considered – because *Borrelia* as a cause cannot be released.

The universe of Internet participants and citizen-scientists has not yet agreed upon the separation of Lyme Disease and co-infections. Thus, everything falls under the term #Lyme Disease, regardless of whether or not Lyme Disease is truly the underlying infection. Patients often find it hard enough to educate others about Lyme Disease; they have all but given up trying to illustrate the differences between Bartonella, Babesia, Ehrlichiosis, etc. It is simpler and easier to connect on the Internet with other affected patients and caregivers by simply using the hashtag #Lyme. Recently, we have heard some use the term 'Lyme-onella.'

When patients don't get better, rather than considering other mechanisms of disease or other important germs, they think **post-hoc** about what property of *Borrelia* can be additionally ascribed to it, then rationalize why it is so evasive in terms of diagnosis and treatment and thereby, justify more useless treatments.

I have heard physicians in lectures say *Borrelia* has a very large genome and many plasmids so it actually has more DNA code to be smarter and more evasive of treatment: some have said *Borrelia* is more like a parasite because it has much more genetic information than any other bacterium. While this may all be true it does not necessarily mean it changes the biology of what *Borrelia* does and it does not necessarily turn it into some sort of a stealthy evasive germ. It is far simpler and more logical to consider that *Borrelia* may not be the cause of the symptoms that don't respond.

If you understand the biological process underlying the disease, then you can stop thinking of *Borrelia* as this resilient germ that can withstand any treatment you throw at it. My experience has indicated the success rates of therapy and the patients' responses are considerably better when you use the correct biological models and testing to think about the disease.

CHRONIC INFECTIONS CAUSE SMALL VESSEL DISEASE

DR. MOZAYENI

The Biology of Chronic Infections

Any chronic inflammatory condition can affect small vessel (micro-vascular) flow to different parts of the brain thereby causing mild or moderate cognitive impairment and sometimes even more severe and overt neurological symptoms. This is all consistent with simply understanding that with a chronic infection there is inflammation, hypercoagulability, and small-vessel disease, limiting blood flow.

Through the understanding of the biology, understanding of the testing, and understanding of the evidence base, there are clearly paths that can be taken to move forward. The new diagnostic tests illuminating this problem better not only identify *Borrelia* better but they can identify other microbes more effectively, as well.

The world is full of microbes. If you look hard enough you will find hundreds if not thousands of chronically present microbes in every individual. The challenge is to know when persistent infections are actually causing the symptoms the patient describes.

Currently, the most accurate method we have to diagnose small-vessel disease is by clinical exam. Even if you could diagnose *Borrelia* (or other co-infections) 100 percent of the time, you still are left with the technological inability to connect the persistence of the infection with the actual symptoms and clinical signs the patient has or with the other inflammatory markers you see on a blood test. The general inflammatory markers one normally looks at are usually not positive in Lyme Disease.

We have been in situations where we have had proof of *Bartonella* in a patient who was completely asymptomatic. And we have had proof of *Protozoa* of different kinds in a patient who was asymptomatic.

The host response variability add much complexity — disease may often be the result of how an individual responds mentally and physically to a germ.

In other words, what is the relative contribution to disease by the germ relative to the host response? No social network would tell you so; thus, patients' sharing notes on these things are usually misleading.

Germ Theory of Disease

Louis Pasteur and his colleague Antoine Beauchamp had the same debate over this issue. On his deathbed, Pasteur conceded to Beauchamp he was right - that, it is the 'terrain' (host response) that defines the disease rather than the microbe.

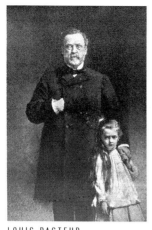
LOUIS PASTEUR

Missing here is the science of how a given individual responds to a germ and how different individuals respond to the same germ. This has been known for decades in the context of streptococcal infections and rheumatic fever. I have seen this clearly in Lyme Disease because recently, we acquired a reliable test for *Bartonella*. I have seen situations where we found *Bartonella* in a patient who became asymptomatic after managing their endocrine issues, for example, their thyroid metabolism problems. I do think these patients need treatment but may do well with a very different kind of treatment than intense regimens of antibiotics.

With a patient who has the infection but no symptoms, one might use a gentler approach, maybe use some herbal supplements that naturally suppress the number of germs to below the threshold at which they would cause a reaction in the body. That threshold is called quorum sensing.

This new microbiological theory suggests that below a critical threshold, bacteria may not have a "quorum" to act in a manner to cause disease. It implies that if you reduce bacteria levels to below the threshold concentration for quorum sensing, they may not cause a disease response by the host.

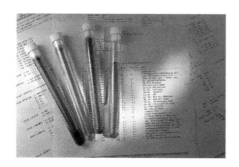

Testing will never be perfect. If a practitioner follows a clinical approach in which the patient's need comes first, my belief is the patient will always do better. Practicing medicine is clinical no matter how good your tests are. You need someone who can explain to the person what is going on, both allaying their fears and understanding the biology of the person's symptoms and disease.

A physician usually understands and appreciates this and Lyme patients are increasingly appreciating and understanding that the best strategy is clinical. But most patients' natural tendency is to believe a diagnostic test more than their clinician, even experienced patients who get treated for Lyme Disease. If you know the caveats of diagnostic testing you will learn to realize there are some tests you should truly believe and there are some you simply cannot believe, one way or the other depending on the clinical circumstances.

The clinical circumstances provide the all-important context for interpretation and action. With the expansion of HMOs, guidelines, and the increasing federalization of health care, physician judgment, clinical context, and patient preference are increasingly less likely to be considered as the national health care agenda shifts from evidence-based medicine to cost control. Eventually, precision, personalied medicine empowered by data should prevail.

Today, the words "evidence-based medicine" may be code for cost-control and rationing of care, confusing 'absence of evidence' with 'evidence of absence.'

SHARON

It's important to look at both clinical symptoms and results of the diagnostic testing. The physician and patient need to assess which tests are clearly defining and accurate and which are superfluous information. If you present with joint pain, low-grade fever, fatigue, and a doctor says your ELISA test was negative and therefore you are not sick, you know you need to find a new physician.

DR. MOZAYENI

The new awareness of small-vessel disease represents a fundamental shift in the core paradigm of Lyme Disease that is essential to advancing treatments.

I am hearing from colleagues who are treating patients with these conditions. They are also noticing *Bartonella* and *Protozoa* seem to play a bigger role in "#Lyme Disease diagnosis" than expected. If so, in some, *Borrelia* may be the co-infection.

We need to stop thinking of *Borrelia* as the ultimate stealth pathogen. We need to understand better the biological process underlying the disease.

If you understand the biological process then you can stop thinking of *Borrelia* as this resilient pathogen that can withstand any treatment you throw at it.

My experience has been that the success rates of therapy and the patients' responses are considerably better when you use the right biological models to think about the disease process.

SMALL VESSEL DISEASE

What is Small Vessel Disease?

If you look carefully at the biology of the Lyme and co-infecting microbes you realize they differ in their potential to cause small-vessel disease. While *Bartonella* co-infection tend to cause more vascular symptoms, *Borrelia* tends **not** to be in the vascular system. You may find it in blood, but we know it likes to get out of the vascular system and get into other tissues, bind collagen, and get into joint linings. Bartonella does this too, as we are able to culture it from skin and other tissues but in the 'non vascular' tissues, Bartonella is less symptomatic.

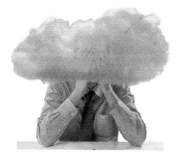

Some of the symptoms patients often have are neurological or neuropsychiatric. The neurological symptoms include those related to central nervous system – poor cognitive function, anxiety, impaired thought processing, mood issues, mood swings, sudden onset of anxiety, rage, and a wide variety of other related issues.

I had no idea my cognitive issues were caused by bacteria. I thought I was not as bright as others, "slow," irritable, moody, and highly anxious. I never knew bacteria could cause my psychiatric issues. My husband experienced the Lyme rage. The proof was in the pudding on this one. Time did tell. Now, my anxiety is almost nil. My auditory processing is not great, but I can create a company budget again, I pay bills on time, I can find the words to describe something. My husband no longer experiences those inexplicable fits of anger.

Recognizing Small Vessel Disease

Small-vessel disease can affect any and all functions of the nervous system. Thorough understanding of blood flow to nervous tissues is essential to being able to diagnose small-vessel disease. A practitioner has to be able to do a thorough neurological exam looking at the subtle features of neurological disease and not only the obvious ones like a stroke. It is the exceptional neurologist who can actually do this which is why it often does not get diagnosed properly.

There are certain features one can look for but it is important to look at the overall picture of the patient's case with regard to the multitude of neurological and neurovascular manifestations.

Psychiatric manifestations can also help to discern whether or not someone has small-vessel disease. To put it differently, looking at the neurological exam that way or completing a neurological exam with attention to such detail gives the practitioner a sensor and trip wire system for detecting small-vessel disease. There are multiple explanations in the biology of these infections and inflammation that explain the psychiatric manifestations.

How Do We Find Small Vessel Disease?

Currently, we do not have a good practical test for looking at the cells lining the blood vessels and we don't have a good test for diagnosing small-vessel disease – an important core feature of this entire disease process that is just simply not thought of or noticed by 'modern medicine.' We do have indirect ways of looking at it, involving biopsies and immuno-staining. A dermatology research scientist at the University of Minnesota, Marna Ericson,

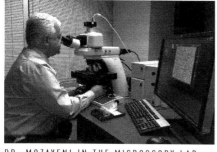

PhD, has shown by fluorescent immuno-staining skin biopsies and subsequent analysis by single- and multi-photon laser scanning microscopy, that *Bartonella* spp. can be detected in normal non-lesional skin.

DR. MOZAYENI IN THE MICROSCOPY LAB

With fluorescent immuno-staining we have learned *Bartonella* are present in and around blood vessels that feed nerves and is not associated with nerves.

This suggests that peripheral nerve symptoms result from small-vessel disease. **It is also possible that chemical signals generated by the Bartonellae or by the infected host would affect peripheral nerves.**

This has led me to think that everything called 'neuro-Lyme' may actually be *Bartonella* or other infections that cause neurological symptoms by primarily affecting blood flow – that *Borrelia* does not like to go into areas (just like any microbe) where there is a low level of nutrition.

At a 2007 ILADS (International Lyme and Associated Diseases) conference in Philadelphia, there was a talk given by Diego Cadavid, M.D., from Rutgers (http://www.ncbi.nlm.nih.gov/pubmed/10908149). In the lab, Cadavid had given monkeys *Borrelia* infections and was showing slides of their brain tissue. As hard he tried, he could not find *Borrelia* in their brain tissue (parenchyma). I lo did, however, find the microbes in the tissues surrounding the brain such as in the leptomeninges, nerve roots, and dorsal root ganglia.

Blood Viscosity

In addition to small-vessel disease you can have infections that increase blood viscosity. For example, significant sludging of blood flow can occur by having the common cold; the inflammation activates platelets, the infection activates platelets, the platelets cause sludging, and the white cells are activated, which then makes the white cells stickier. The stickier the cells become, the greater the flow is diminished through the capillaries because they stick to the wall of the capillary and the red cells move through sluggishly. This is part of the body's defense system to try to wall off the spread of germs throughout the body.

DR. MOZAYENI

In a patient with chronic infection, this process happens constantly but regionally and then, in cycles. There are parts of the body and elements of the biochemistry of the blood where clots are forming and dissolving, all the time.

Thus, some parts of the body may be exhibiting symptoms while other parts may be asymptomatic.

SHARON

This makes sense to me. It took eight minutes to draw one vial of blood before I started seeing Dr. Mozayeni. My blood looked like thick mucous. When I asked the phlebotomist why it was like that, she shook her head and said, "I don't know." I kept thinking, "If it's that thick in my arm, it's that thick trying to go through my heart..." I couldn't help but wonder why I hadn't suffered a heart attack or stroke. But no one seemed too concerned about the thickness of the blood except it took them longer to collect the specimen for the testing.

DR. MOZAYENI

How Does Bartonella Play into the Small Vessel Disease Picture?

How practitioners evaluate and treat patients is evolving as we consider the role of chronic infections. That *Bartonella* is primarily a vascular infection helps us reframe the issueappreciating that perhaps *Borrelia* is not necessarily the biggest cause of the symptoms in patients with Lyme Disease. Knowing *Bartonella* is a vascular infection helps us to make a very important paradigm shift:

Perhaps *Borrelia* is NOT necessarily the single cause of the symptoms in patients who test positive for Lyme Disease especially when they have neurologically dominant symptoms.

With small vessel disease in the picture and knowing *Bartonella* is primarily a vascular infection, I started looking carefully at *Bartonella.* This was in 2008 at a time when there were only very ineffective, insensitive, and inaccurate *Bartonella* tests on the market, even in the best labs.

We knew *Bartonella* was a player in Lyme Disease but we could not know when and where and how it was a player and in which patients.

Since medical school, I have had an interest in vascular inflammation, beginning when I was a researcher in the transplantation immunology lab of the Department of Surgery at Albany Medical College. There, I learned when organs are rejected in a transplant it is because there is an immune reaction to the lining of the blood vessels of the transplanted organ. It is not white cells going in and damaging the tissue of the organ; the white blood cells react to the vessel lining and this process blocks the blood flow.

We also know *Bartonella* is primarily an endovascular infection. *Bartonella* is a germ that likes to stay in your vascular system because it likes the iron in hemoglobin. Hemoglobin is a protein with a center chemical root called heme and at the center of that is iron and cobalt.

The *Bartonella* like heme and oxygen. They like to stay in the vascular system. If you look at it from the point of view of the bacteria, the vascular system is the area of the body most rich in oxygen and nutrients.

While *Bartonella* is primarily an endovascular infection, it has also been known to cause infection of the endothelial cell that line blood vessels; not only the red cells and the blood components.

This is what is lost on most of the medical system. We draw blood and we look at things in blood but we don't draw out and inspect the cells lining the blood vessels.

If you don't see some microbes in the blood that you draw, you would never know if there is an infection of the lining of the blood vessels.

How Does Inflammation Complicate Chronic Infections?

With inflammation coming from chronic infections, you get disruption of capillary flow, not only from inflammation and the stickiness of white cells but also because your coagulation system becomes activated and this thickens your blood. Often when you cannot see markers of inflammation with these chronic infections you can see coagulation disorders. For example, the CRP is often normal or slightly elevated and so your usual inflammatory markers fail you. Some inflammatory markers may be affected however when those regular markers fail you and you may not believe there is a chronic infection.

But if you look at the coagulation system using very good tests with the blood specimens drawn, carefully, properly handled and sent out quickly on dry ice to the lab, you can actually see evidence of hyper-coagulation. When you do see evidence of hyper-coagulation, you then realize we are also dealing with yet another component of these chronic conditions, hyper-coagulation that affects the flow at the capillary level. In lay terms, hyper-coagulation is called blood thickening.

The coagulation system is really a polymer network. Fibrin monomers link together to form fibrin polymers, which constitute the majority of a blood clot. In the clot, you can get both germs and cells trapped inside. Thus, the major point: when you have clumps of stuff forming and little clots in the circulation and on the inside of the blood vessels you essentially have what some people are now beginning to notice as biofilm.

Bio-films

The topic of biofilm is very hot in some disciplines like pharmacokinetics where they are looking at it as a potentially very important factor in the effectiveness of antibiotic therapy, as well as chemotherapy. For three years now, I have been studying biofilms in our clinical CLIA-certified lab on every patient.

We are developing new methods to measure how much biofilm a patient may have in their circulation. This capability does not exist elsewhere. You might be able to get a picture of a piece of biofilm here and there on a blood smear but there is no way to quantitate it for me to know how much of a biofilm load there is as I take care of a patient. So much of a patient's symptoms are due directly to the burden of the biofilm.

Germ Response Variability

Because of the emphasis on small-vessel disease, we have to look also at blood coagulation, which then relates also to coagulation genetics. Ultimately, this gets into a discussion of host response. You can have one germ causing completely different diseases in different people – this is because genes that affect the immune and coagulation responses vary among individuals.

The classic example is chronic streptococcus: some people get cardiac dominant rheumatic fever, some get arthritis dominant rheumatic fever. Now we see some kids get PANDAS (Pediatric

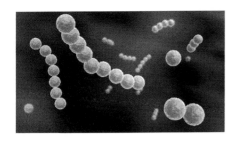

Autoimmune Neuropsychiatric Disorders Associated with Streptococcal Infections). If you have one manifestation you tend not to get the other – that they are mutually exclusive. This is due to variability in the immune-genetic response.

The coagulation system is also genetically variable. You have people with predispositions to having thick blood or thin blood and those with naturally thinner blood may develop less intense symptoms or not develop symptoms as severe as those who have genetic predispositions.

There may be other host response factors affecting the circulatory system. For example, the endothelial cells may proliferate more intensely in one patient than in another patient. It depends on, for example, how sensitive the endothelial cell is to the hormones coming from the platelets, that may stick to the vessel lining, because the infection is there. Knowing this would take you down a different pathway of how you manage the patient's care.

Simply, we are scientifically at the beginning of the process of trying to understand the relative contribution of the germ versus the host to the resulting disease. It is important to realize the disease is a net reaction of:

- the germ

- the host
- nutrition
- environment
- stress levels, and
- even the mind, body, and spiritual state of the individual.

All of the above listed is what determines how the disease ultimately manifests and what you do about it; different in every one, yet patients want so much to publicize their wish to receive the 'one size fits all protocol.'

Patients are looking for everyone else's experiences to guide and validate them in ways that cannot possibly occur, because the host response is so highly variable.

Considering Small Vessel Disease During Diagnosis

The small-vessel disease concept is one that can be lost on the medical system, Lyme-literate doctors included; mostly, because there is not a good test for it. Doctors are not being taught to look for it. An appreciation of the vascular biology, good clinical judgment and a good 'sub-cortical' neurological exam are required to know when small vessel disease is present.

Vascular impairment can in leave some permanent damage, small vessel disease usually won't. It usually leaves behind injured tissue. In the nervous system, there may be dysfunctional, stunned or

DR. MOZAYENI

hibernating nerves. This concept is well established in cardiology were heart muscle may be compromised by poor blood flow.

Many neurologists still believe nerves are either fully functional or they are completely dead and there is nothing in between. Nothing in the entire body resembles this, so the notion that a nerve would be like that is ridiculous – nerves can be idling or dysfunctional. But many neurologists and neuroscientists, to this day, would be unnerved by this rupture of their paradigm.

Many people, including physicians, tend to see the world in black and white. They can be binary in their thinking process. The small-vessel disease concept is very helpful because it is actually the scientific way to think about the problem. This opens the door up to a few different interesting scenarios about how you manage it and where you place your priorities in terms of what microbes you are looking at and what to focus on.

If physicians consider small vessel disease, they would be more likely to appropriately consider infections that are largely within the vascular system as the primary suspects – i.e., *Bartonella* or *Protozoa* rather than *Borrelia*. Knowing the biology of these organisms redirects attention more appropriately, especially when neurological symptoms are dominant features in a case.

*Protozoa*n infections, like *Babesia* and *Protomyxzoa,* have similarities to other known *Protozoa* infections like malaria. These too are infections of the vascular system.

If one sees a lot of small-vessel disease, it is usually predominantly an endovascular infection and then it can be assumed **Bartonella and/or *Protozoa* play a dominant role. These germs infect the vessels that also feed the nervous system and they may cause more neuro-psychiatric manifestations.**

In a patient with neurovascular manifestations, I now tend to think we are dealing usually with *Bartonella* and *Protozoa* principally and that *Borrelia* may have a smaller role. The central nervous system has specially adapted transport systems to get nutrients from the blood vessels to the nerves and this makes it harder for microbes to invade the central nervous system. But these microbes do certainly impair brain blood flow in a patchy, regional, and fluctuating manner.

When *Borrelia* is present, it tends to be associated with joint pain and sometimes joint swelling, perhaps because the lining of the joints (synovium) is very vascular; it is getting its nourishment from the vessels of connective tissue. That is why there may often be a lot of symptoms related to synovial inflammation associated with chronic infections, *Bartonella* and *Protozoa* included.

Given some of these new perspectives, the question then becomes: How does this realization shift the diagnostic and therapeutic emphasis? We have covered this briefly:

- You have to look at *Bartonella* with the best available test.
- You have to look at the *Protozoa* with the best available test, and
- You have to understand: **It is a far stronger form of evidence when you have molecular proof of these various Lyme-related infections using these new tests than having a few antibody bands on a Western blot.**

We need to use molecular tests to succeed more with our therapies.

BACTERIA
CAUSES PAIN

SHARON

I'm including this information because when I read it, it gave me a tremendous sense of validation for the pain I have experienced over the past three decades. The article does not pertain to Lyme directly, but it does promise to lead to more discoveries eventually helping chronically ill patients.

DR. MOZAYENI

There was a study published in *Nature Magazine*, the most prominent scientific journal there is. Published on September 5, 2013, this paper explains how bacteria can directly activate sensory neurons that modulate pain and inflammation. We have unexplained pain syndromes in many patients with chronic infections. Until now we have been postulating the pain is due to some damage that occurs, falsely triggering pain fibers. It can also affect sensory fibers or motor fibers that can cause numbness and tingling or weakness in a muscle. But now we know they can directly modulate pain.

We don't know which bacteria could do this but this article lays out how it is highly plausible and to expect that bacteria can do this. This explains why some pain treatments haven't been effective and it might even explain why some of the pain that increases during treatment is probably because some of these characteristics might be enhanced during the course of treatment.

In medical school, we were all trained and taught the epidermis, the dead layer of skin on the surface, actually doesn't have anything living in it. We knew it doesn't have blood vessels, but we assumed it didn't have nerve endings either. Well, it turns out even though it is dead skin tissue it does have living nerve endings. Remember, nerves transport nutrients through the nerve body, through the neuron, so the nerve tips can extend into the epidermis and be fed through the neuron itself. Those nerve endings don't need to have blood flow – they are fed by the nerve itself.

TRANSIENT
SYMPTOMS

Vascular flow issues may explain why patients get transient symptoms. They may get a transient neurological problem or a transient muscular problem that may appear to be 'migrating.' The germ is not moving around; rather the flow may be fluctuating at a microscopic level in different tissues at different times.

Small vessel disease in a patient is like having little local 'brown outs' in the electrical grid all the time. You have these micro-level little 'brown outs' happening all the time and thus, a general reduction of overall capillary flow systemically resulting in people having much reduced stamina and much reduced energy.

What is Peripheral Neuropathy?

There is also the potential to have peripheral nerve problems, including fluctuating or episodic numbness or tingling. This can include false vibratory sensations and also, of course, pain.

Each type of sensation is carried by a different nerve in the body. How these things are affected may have something to do with how much myelin these nerves have.

We have to remember a nerve is a very, very long single cell. It is the longest cell in the body. It can be even a few microns wide while at the same time being a meter long, which means it is going to need a blood supply along its entire pathway.

If you have a long wire and a whole bunch of people with wire cutters coming at it, you are more likely to lose that circuit. Very simply: long wires, i.e. long nerves, are more vulnerable to a random inflammatory process in the body that affects the small blood vessels because long nerves present a bigger target.

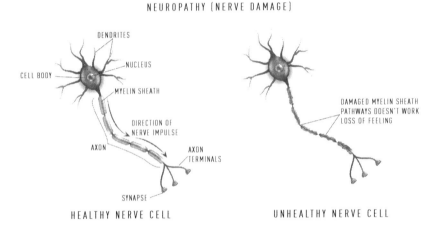

NEUROPATHY (NERVE DAMAGE)

DENDRITES

NUCLEUS

CELL BODY

MYELIN SHEATH

DIRECTION OF
NERVE IMPULSE

AXON

AXON
TERMINALS

SYNAPSE

HEALTHY NERVE CELL

DAMAGED MYELIN SHEATH
PATHWAYS DOESN'T WORK
LOSS OF FEELING

UNHEALTHY NERVE CELL

A peripheral nerve, or the spinal cord, or the brain, has a deep blood supply that usually has a lot of redundancy of blood flow pathways. We refer to these as collateral flow pathways. The gray matter of the central nervous system has much collateral blood flow, however, the deep white matter areas have limited collateral flow channels and are more vulnerable to small vessel disease. These white matter areas are the interconnecting 'wires' and thus, their compromise often causes neuro-psychiatric and cognitive symptoms.

In the peripheral nervous system there is a blood supply to the entire length of the nerve but it is not one blood supply. It comes from many regional arteries along its course.

Nerves, arteries, and veins travel together in the body so it is possible that branches of an artery that are near a nerve feed it along its course. But if the small vessels at the capillary level that feed the nerve are being injured or blocked at different points along its path, it can potentially disrupt the entire path.

Throughout the body, you have micro-level 'brown outs' happening all the time and a general reduction of overall capillary flow, which gives patients much reduced stamina and energy. Symptoms vary greatly depending on what tissue or area of tissue involved by this process.

Other kinds of nerves that can be affected are those that control the autonomic nervous system. That includes nerves that regulate the vagal tone of the body, which lowers your heart rate and allows you to relax.

POTS (Postural Orthostatic Tachycardia Syndrome)

The emergency or 'fight or flight' side of the autonomic nervous system is activated by stress and mediated by adrenaline. Those nervous systems also can have interruptions of blood flow but they have a very different manifestation. A patient may tend to have problems with blood pressure control or a rapid heartbeat. Some of these patients are given the diagnosis of POTS (Postural Orthostatic Tachycardia Syndrome) and are often managed with beta-blockers to minimize the fluctuations of their adrenaline-related symptoms. I have also had patients who have had this managed using drugs that are used to treat myasthenia gravis. ***POTS is a condition often associated with and likely caused by chronic infections.***

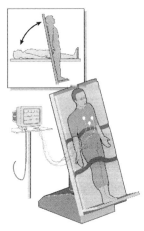

HEAD-UP TILT TABLE (HUT) TESTING IS THE STANDARD METHOD TO ASSESS A PATIENT'S REACTION TO POSTURAL CHANGE. THIS INVOLVES PLACING THE PATIENT ON THE TILT TABLE, AND MEASURING BLOOD PRESSURE AND HEART RATE. THEN THE TABLE IS TILTED UPRIGHT TO A 60-80 DEGREE VERTICAL ANGLE FOR APPROXIMATELY 45 MIN AND BLOOD PRESSURE AND HEART RATE ARE AGAIN MEASURED, EITHER CONTINUOUSLY, OR AT LEAST EVERY 2-3 MIN

WHY TESTING FOR CO-INFECTIONS IS CRITICAL FOR SUCCESSFUL TREATMENT

DR. MOZAYENI

Limited Testing Options

When I first started my search for better co-infection testing, my training as a medical scientist was very helpful. Having worked in the research lab and having run Western blots myself, I was familiar with the caveats of the test. I know how messy the blots can look when you are done. I know how hard it can be to interpret them. I also have put these blots through automated scanning systems that attempt to quantitate the bands and I know how potentially inaccurate those automated scans can be.

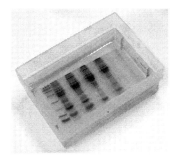

When I looked at the whole landscape of what diagnostic tests were available, in my mind, I scored them in terms of my confidence level about the result they would give. When I looked at *Borrelia* Western blots I gave it sort of a 3 or 4 out of 10 in terms of how confident I would be in the result if I saw a positive. There are some Western blots so glaringly positive that no one would argue them. That is part of the problem with the test. The result produced is along a spectrum of potential levels of confidence with great variability of clinical context. You can have a couple of weak bands and to a really sick patient with no other answers - those results can justify their treatment. To a healthy patient, the same results would be interpreted as negative or normal. Context is always important, not only for interpretation of test results, but for choice and timing of treatment. This is rooted in mathematics, not professional opinion and is called 'predictive value.'

Great – but what if you get the wrong treatment because you have *Bartonella* causing weak positive bands on the *Borrelia* Western blot? Then you are going to have only a temporary improvement and a relapse. Then Lyme doctors will start telling you "we can temporarily get you better but we cannot fix you." Usually, as much as they may try, they don't actually know the cause; or they do know and may not have the right treatment.

If you see only IgM-positive bands on the Lyme Western blot, you definitely need to test for co-infections, especially Bartonella.

The *Borrelia* Western blot scores a 3 or 4 out of 10 in terms of my general confidence level because it is an indirect test, looking at antibody responses to a germ. There is nothing better than actually directly detecting a germ such as by detecting its DNA signature or at least its unique proteins encoded by the DNA. Then you can be sure you have that microbe. Unfortunately, a sensitive and specific test like this has not been available for *Borrelia*. Lately, some companies have developed enrichment culture methods for *Borrelia*. This is encouraging but fraught with pitfalls for potential contamination.

We need more experience with it to know how confident we can be. It depends on the actual laboratory technique they use to detect it, how they confirm that what they find is really *Borrelia,* and the precautions taken to prevent contamination. They need to do full genetic sequencing to confirm. But if *Borrelia burgdorferi* has such a huge genome, while challenging, it will become much easier very soon to sequence the full genome of every isolate of *Borrelia* found in culture.

In 2008, we had more limited testing. As of Fall of 2011 we have a commercially available *Bartonella* test. We also now have a commercially available *Babesia* FISH test considered to be sensitive for *Babesia* for DNA detection. We now have better tests (in my opinion) for *Bartonella* and *Protozoa* than we actually have for *Borrelia*. So we have gone from a dearth of tests for *Bartonella* and *Protozoa* to having better labs than those available for *Borrelia*. Recently, better *Borrelia* tests, such as the Nanotrap® Lyme Antigen (LA) Test, have arrived.

If you are tracking antibody changes on a Western blot, it can be helpful to use a test that gives you a measure of the intensity for each band. A more sensitive measure may produce false positives but it can help follow the changes over time. The IGeneX sensitive and semi-quantitative Western blot has been helpful this way.

Other Western blot providers including SUNY Stony Brook, provide you with the other bands if they are positive. They will tell you if you have bands 31 and 34 even though they are not the 'approved' bands because 31 and 34 are specific to *Borrelia*. It is good to know if these antibodies are present.

Interestingly, Stony Brook does not tell you their test is negative unless every band is negative. They usually tell you it is indeterminate if it is not clearly positive. Scientifically, they are saying you cannot really use this test to say *Borrelia* is not there. Large commercial labs do not test bands 31 and 34 and they do report results as negative making false negative results more likely.

There are definitely some *caveats,* but again my confidence level in the *Borrelia* Western blot, on a scale of 10, is 3-4, or strongly positive, with all of the bands, a 9. Depending on the result my confidence level in the test would vary. This is not a reliable test characteristic because you are always trying to recalibrate the result in your head and explain it to the patient and incorporate that probabilistic assessment in your patient care. In other words, it is a method that yields ambiguous results that would support almost any clinical decision unless strongly positive or strongly negative.

Finding a Reliable Bartonella Test

In 2007, I researched any and all available *Bartonella* tests. Basically, there were only antibody tests using commercial kits, which were available from major labs for only two species of *Bartonella*. The kit had been distributed years earlier, so it probably went through FDA approval for strains of *Bartonella* that may actually be out of date and/or vary in their prevalence. Hardly anyone was turning up positive on this test (in my experience) yet we knew *Bartonella* to be a common co-infection.

We also went to a major lab, which at the time had a special test for culturing hard-to-grow organisms called the fastidious gram-negative rod culture.

In the same time frame, the test from Dr. Breitschwerdt's research lab at NC State showed 20 percent positive in the first set of patients we started testing. None of the other labs showed any positive results - not a single positive. My general sense of the value of the existing *Bartonella* testing out there, for the antibody testing, was less than a 1 out of 10; for the commercial *Bartonella* culture test available at that time, we never even turned up one positive result.

This test failure occurred in a group later shown in our published research to be as high as 60% positive. Not even *one* positive result was seen in any *Bartonella* testing platform - **ZERO**. There was no commercially available *Bartonella* culture detection system at all, in the United States as of 2008.

For the *Protozoa* we had the *Babesia* FISH tests, but we did not have a test for any other *Protozoa* because they were still in the process of being discovered. *Protomyxzoa rheumatica* PR just got its name in the summer of 2011. There was no molecular test for *PR* until shortly after that point.

We have to recognize with all microbe groups that they are part of a spectrum. To think about individual germs with individual names is really not scientifically accurate. We have to think of *Bartonella* variants, we have to think of *Protozoa* variants, we have to think of *Borrelia* variants, and there are probably other germs too, like different forms of *Mycoplasma, Anaplasma*, etc.

In our veterinarian human patients, the people who provide medical care for animals, when they get cultured for *Bartonella*, they tend to have more growth of the *Bartonella* because they have not been already treated with a variety of different antibiotics; whereas our Lyme patients tend not to show growth, making their *Bartonella* harder to detect. The *Bartonella* is more difficult to detect because they have been through other treatments or they are on protocols that are not really working but can suppress the microbe.

We also have been testing patients in the research lab for other infections like *Mycoplasma.* Our non-veterinarian patients tend not to have that. The veterinarians tend to have a higher rate of *Mycoplasma*, again probably because they have not been treated or they are more exposed. Veterinarians are a more high-risk individual profession, usually untreated when diagnosed, as opposed to a chronic Lyme patient who has had risk factors but has also been on a lot of different medications.

Benefits of Better Testing

By working with a better *Bartonella* test since 2008, I have been able to clinically experience the benefit of the test and to realize through clinical care that it does fit with the theory of small-vessel disease. This gets into how the awareness of small-vessel disease changes the approach to therapy. Not only does it change the focus on a germ but it also makes one consider other aspects of vascular health, disease, and circulation.

For example, could *Bartonella* be causing proliferation of the endothelium (the thin layer of cells that lines the interior surface of blood vessels and lymphatic vessels)? If it does, it needs to be researched further because infection of the vascular lining is usually the first step in the development and progression of arteriosclerosis.

In the future, we will have to see if *Bartonella* is actually one of the causes of arteriosclerosis. I think it is likely that we will eventually

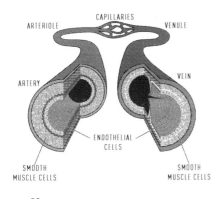

ARTERIOLE CAPILLARIES VENULE
ARTERY VEIN
ENDOTHELIAL CELLS
SMOOTH MUSCLE CELLS SMOOTH MUSCLE CELLS

find it does contribute often to classic arteriosclerotic vascular disease.

Good lab testing is very important because there are ways of knowing how you know; it's a heuristic approach. You have to know what is there before you know if what you are doing is actually working on what you know is there. If you do not know what is there and just wing it because you have this clinical defined notion of what the problem is based on general symptoms, then you may not be really be applying the best treatments. One has to know the microbiology, immunology and be very analytical.

For example, we are finding other *Protozoa* cause false positive results on some *Babesia* tests.

You have to understand enough immunology to know how that is possible. Then you treat what you think is really there and watch to see if the cross-reacting antibody to *Babesia* actually goes away. But if you try a specific *Babesia* treatment the *Babesia* antibody doesn't go away because it may actually be a cross-reacting antibody to a different germ. Unless you are really careful to observe the data and understand the immunology you will miss it.

Another example: when you have any infection, particularly one that causes low-grade smoldering inflammation and immune suppression, like a *Bartonella*, you can produce lots of immunoglobulin M (IgM), a less specific large five molecule cluster antibody that is an early phase antibody. Because it is not a very specific antibody, it will tend to cross react on IgM tests for other microbes. So if one has IgM to a microbe they are going to tend to get IgMs to other microbes.

We have seen a number of cases where the patient had *Bartonella* proven by culture and confirmed by DNA sequencing, but then had only IgM to *Borrelia*, which is what could be interpreted as having evidence for *Borreliosis*, aka Lyme Disease. There are many, many, many patients who think they have Lyme Disease because they have IgM to *Borrelia* but the IgM could have been cross-reacting to *Bartonella*. You sometimes cannot be sure at the point of starting treatment. But if you follow those antibodies, you will often find that those IgM antibodies go away with the treatment of the other infection.

If you are looking for evidence of *Borrelia* you expect more and more IgG and less IgM to be produced as you treat the infection. **If you don't get any IgG production on a Western blot for *Borrelia* as you treat for it, then you probably were not dealing with *Borrelia* in the first place** unless the patient has a major other reason to be immune suppressed.

All of these subtleties are reminders: you have to keep looking for the core problem and the host responses.

If you do not test for co-infections you do not know what you are treating.

You don't know where to put the emphasis of your treatment. Many LLMDs don't employ the latest testing for co-infections.

A number of different prominent physicians who treat Lyme patients are saying if you don't deal with the co-infections first, then it is going to be a lot harder to treat *Borrelia.*

Another way to interpret this: a lot of Lyme-like symptoms may be from these other infections and it is not really Lyme Disease (i.e., caused by *Borrelia* spp).

> **_Bartonella_ is and can be a co-infection of _Borrelia_**
> **but there are so many ways to contract _Bartonella_**
> **than there are ways to get _Borrelia_.**

As we learn more and more about *Bartonella,* I am convinced we are going to find this is relatively common. It is a microbe that infects all mammals to the point where it may be so prevalent that we don't even notice it because it becomes part of the normal landscape causing many common chronic diseases.

Disease Transmission to Humans

There are many ways to get *Bartonella*, including from your cat. When infected, cats have about a 500,000x higher circulating level of *Bartonella*. If they are indoor/outdoor cats or feral cats, 80% or more carry *Bartonella*. The numbers are probably higher but even the sickest cats will have a few consecutive days of the month during which they will have no detectable *Bartonella* in their blood.

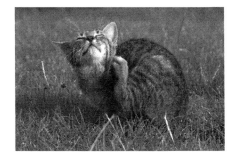

There are many ways to get *Bartonella*: from fleas, cats, and potentially other biting insects strongly suspected but not strictly proven. So it is likely a much more prevalent infection.

The other *Protozoa* infections probably follow the same pathways in terms of the ways they are spread. Vectors are agents that transmit the various *Protozoa* that makes people sick. *Protozoa* get into and on red cells that can be transmitted by mosquitoes, known transmitters of *Protozoa*. It stands to reason, then, that *Babesia* and *Babesia*-like microbes can be transmitted by mosquitoes.

Here we all are worried about deer ticks and most patients with Lyme Disease cannot remember a deer tick bite. But everyone I know can remember a mosquito bite. Everyone I know has probably run into fleas more often than they have run into deer ticks. There are all kinds of fleas. There are sand fleas at the beach. There are fleas on your cat, fleas on your dog.

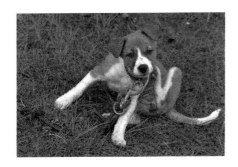

Nine percent of dogs carry *Bartonella* but when they do, their blood levels are a lot lower so I don't think they represent as big a reservoir or a risk as cats do.

The landscape of chronic infection is far bigger than just *Borrelia*.

This probably explains why patients with these chronic symptoms tend to classify their condition as "Lyme Disease"; it punches their card into a support system. It is a way to describe what they have. **But using the term "Lyme Disease" retards scientific progress because the term is too broad, given the way it is used by the layperson and even many LLMDs.**

SHARON

I recently attended a Lyme-related conference and listened as two well-respected physicians stated they believe the primary "culprit" to treat in chronically ill patients is *Borrelia*.

These two physicians who spoke at the conference stated they rarely test for co-infections. After spending so many years trying to figure out what was causing my symptoms, I couldn't help but think,

If you do not <u>look</u> for something,
you are probably not going to <u>find</u> it.

It is true that only a short time ago testing for co-infections was not

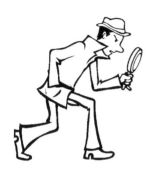

very accurate, but medical science continues to make amazing, significant discoveries in this field. When I started treatment in September of 2009, these tests were not yet available.

Maybe most patients do have Lyme and not a co-infection. But we certainly will never find out unless all patients are tested for co-infections from these new, reliable testing facilities.

**My treatment would never have succeeded
if I had not been tested for co-infections.**

Please, get tested for co-infections from the specialty labs. Yes, it is expensive. But the treatment protocol for co-infections will be different than the treatment for *Borrelia*.

You cannot be treated properly if you don't know what infections you have. And if you cannot be treated properly, you will not heal.

Separating Lyme Disease and Bartonella

This is why I make the key point, when I lecture on *Bartonella*, that *Bartonella* is a co-infection of Lyme but it also in and of itself is an infection that may be more prevalent than *Borrelia*. Because a lot of its symptoms resemble Lyme, because the Lyme patients are not getting co-infections tested, and because they are obsessed over *Borrelia* and deer ticks to the fault of excluding other possibilities, they end up misplacing the priority, putting the wrong emphasis on the wrong diagnosis and treatment.

The lay definition of Lyme Disease has actually evolved to the point where it is no longer just *Borrelia*. It is everything possibly related to chronic infection that has ever been seen in association with *Borrelia* even though in and of itself some other chronic infection may be the only issue.

I don't know how that is going to evolve, but for the time being, "#Lyme" is a way to communicate a picture about symptoms in social networks trying to figure out what they have. '#Lyme Disease' is not a medically precise term but it greatly helps a patient to be understood and have some hope for solution.

SECTION THREE

DO YOU SEE YOURSELF IN HERE?

"Perception is seeing the present with images formed from the past."

– EDWARD BEAR

SHARON'S SYMPTOM HISTORY

SHARON

I was the typical "List of Symptoms" patient. The simplest way to present my own history to you, the reader, is to show you how many different types of physicians I saw, some of the major medical events that occurred, and of course, the various diagnoses I was assigned. I know many patients can probably relate to this snapshot.

Physicians Sharon Saw For Symptoms

Often, I saw more than one each of the following:

Cardiologist, Chiropractor, Dentist, Dermatologist, Endocrinologist, Gastroenterologist, Gynecologist, Internist, Neurologist, Neurosurgeon, Ophthalmologist, Optometrist, Oral Surgeon, Orthopedist, Osteopath, Otolaryngologist (ENT), Physical Therapist, Psychologist, Psychiatrist, Rheumatologist, Surgeon, Urologist

Sharon's Symptom and Diagnosis History

1981: viral meningitis, unexplained fatigue and exhaustion

1984: diarrhea, abdominal pain, loss of appetite, mouth ulcers, grinding teeth/jaw pain

1988: elevated gastrin levels

1993: depression and anxiety

1995: migraines

1996: H.Pylori infection

1999: shattered right foot

2001: recurrent sinus infections, night sweats, hot flashes, dry skin, itchy ears

2002: falling easily, pain in knees and thighs, muscle weakness, sensitivity to sunlight, memory loss

2003: clumsiness, repeated falls, muscle weakness, thigh pain, swollen joints, tooth dies

2004: gallstones, abdominal pain, fatigue, hair loss, noise sensitivity

2005: gastrin level elevated, depression, forgetfulness, trouble focusing, sticky blood

2006: diarrhea, headaches, daytime sleepiness and insomnia, elevated heart rate, word and name search, phasing out of conversations

2008: persistent, dry cough, numbness in hands and feet, chest pains, muscle twitching

2009: back pain, hip pain, occasional blurry vision, incontinence, unexplained rashes, positive Lupus test (positive ANA with speckled pattern)

Other General Conditions

ALLERGIES: seasonal allergies, chronic sinus infections

CARDIOVASCULAR: low blood pressure, perspire easily, dizzy upon standing

CONSTITUTIONAL: migraines, weight gain, fatigue, cold extremities, afternoon drowsiness, night sweats, sensitivity to chemicals

EARS, NOSE, MOUTH & THROAT: sensitivity to sounds, ringing in the ears, sinusitis, mercury/silver fillings in teeth, mouth ulcers, jaw paint/ teeth grinding, dental problems, unexplained face pain

ENDOCRINE: heat intolerant, cold intolerant, thyroid disorder, low body temperature

EYES & VISION: dry eyes, blurred vision, floating spots, light sensitive, peripheral waves

DIGESTIVE SYSTEM: bloating, trouble digesting fats, hemorrhoids, ulcers, irritable bowel, diarrhea, abdominal pain, nausea/upset stomach

GENITO-URINARY SYSTEM: incontinence, cramps, heavy flow, PMS, menstrual irregularity, menstrual pain, pelvic pain, health fluctuates with cycles, hot flashes

HEMATOLOGICAL: Anemia, leg pain with walking

IMMUNOLOGICAL: autoimmune disease (Lupus)

INTEGUMENTARY: acne, dermatitis, yellow tone, brittle nails, dry/brittle hair, crawling sensation in skin, various rashes, on/off rashes, skin sensitivity, sensitivity to sunlight, hair loss

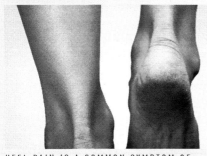

HEEL PAIN IS A COMMON SYMPTOM OF BARTONELLA PATIENTS

MUSCULAR-SKELETAL: back pain, intolerance to exercise, heel pain, disc problems, joint pain and swelling, joint stiffness, bone pain, muscle weakness, muscle twitching/spasm, muscle pain/

cramping, sore soles in the morning, neck stiffness/pain, tremors

NEUROLOGICAL: clumsy, trouble balancing, numbness/tingling, forgetting simple tasks, disorientation/getting lost, difficulty with reading and concentration, speech difficulty, word and name search, memory problems

PSYCHOLOGICAL-BEHAVIORAL: vivid dreams, fearful/worrier, depression, narcolepsy, insomnia, emotional/crying easily, season affective disorder, feeling as though you are losing your mind

RESPIRATORY: shortness of breath, chronic cough, air hungry, snoring, sleep apnea

Other diagnoses given:

Achlorhydria without evidence of Pernicious Anemia, Anxiety, Bursitis, Degenerative Disc Disease, Depression, Dry Eye, Epstein-Barr, Eczema, Gallstones, H.Pylori, Hashimoto's, Herpes Simplex I, Hypo-Thyroidism, Idiopathic Daytime Hypersomnia, Idiopathic Intermittent Right Temporal Waves, Incontinence, Irritable Bowel Syndrome, Lipoma, Migraines, Peri-menopause, Peripheral Neuropathy, Post-Traumatic Stress Disorder, Shingles, Sinusitis, Stomach Antrim Atrophy, Vitamin D Deficiency, Viral Meningitis, Zollinger-Ellison Syndrome possibility

TYPICAL PATIENT
CHARACTERISTICS

Physical Characteristics

Lyme Disease is called "The Great Masquerader," as it mimics so many other diseases. It is not just a bull's eye rash. In fact, up to 60 percent of Lyme patients never even see a rash. When meeting fellow "Lymies" I found there was not really one common denominator in what this disease looks like or how it presents.

Even within my own family, it manifested in three very different forms. My husband Jeff had what would come the closest to "looking like" Lyme Disease. He had a rash on his leg. For two years, he was told it was eczema. Two dermatologists and two internists prescribed various creams. When Dr. Mozayeni saw it, he declared it was certainly not a typical *Borrelia* or *Bartonella* rash, but it certainly was not eczema.

Our son Stephen developed what appeared as "stretch marks" on his trunk and arms. They looked like miniature fireworks with bright red marks at one end. Stephen also suffered from recurrent pneumonia, a low-grade fever, and he tested positive for mononucleosis twice.

The only skin rash I recall is six months before the accurate diagnosis. I developed a rash on my back. The dermatologist swore it was shingles, except it crossed my spinal column, which is impossible for shingles to do. She took five biopsies, including core samples. "Herpes," she declared. "You need to inform your husband."

Lyme manifests in many different forms. It usually appears as illnesses related to autoimmune disorders.

For 29 years, I watched physicians write "auto-immune?" on my chart, never knowing a series of auto-immune diseases could point in the direction of Lyme and its co-infections. I never thought viral meningitis, joint pain, recurrent sinus infections, Hashimoto Syndrome, and itchy ears could be related.

"List of Symptoms" Patients

And then there is the patient who comes in with a very thick file, innumerable diagnoses, and usually very little hope. Most of these patients are women who might have been previously been diagnosed with Chronic Fatigue Syndrome, Fibromyalgia, Lupus,

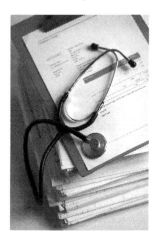

Multiple Sclerosis, depression, anxiety, ALS, Rheumatoid Arthritis, Severe PMS, mood swings, severe anemia, early onset Alzheimer's, peripheral neuropathy, and other neuro-vascular ailments. Many of them have seen between three and twenty sub specialists before getting to a 'Lyme Literate Medical Doctor'.

By the time these patients find the LLMD, they are experiencing feelings of hopelessness and frustration. Some wonder if they are indeed hypochondriacs as family and coworkers might have intimated. Some wonder if they are mentally ill or just plain crazy. They often feel alone, unwanted, disrespected, and damaged.

The fatigue is a very striking feature because they patients are compromised in so many ways that it becomes hard for them to function and they can't get restful sleep; many of them have muscle pain.

By this point, many have lost at least one job due to their illness, either due to the inability even to get into work, or being unable to physically or mentally execute the tasks required for their job. Many patients suffer a loss of executive functioning skills; they find it impossible to prioritize tasks, they have trouble going through piles of paper, organizing their day, balancing their checkbook, even finding their way home.

Financial insecurity usually surfaces between the loss of executive functioning and physical pain and disability. If you don't have a job or you can't pay the bills on time, finances become a worry; not to mention the money spent on medical bills trying to find out what's wrong.

By this point, many friends have fallen out of the picture, often frustrated by the patient's lack of energy to meet for something as simple as coffee or lunch, much less able to stroll the mall or go ice-skating. Friends often tire of hearing the "same old complaints" of the patient's symptoms that never seem to dissipate.

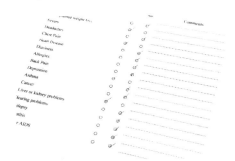

Even as the patient goes from one specialist to another, they might become labeled drug seekers or menopausal. They are often given numerous psychiatric disorder diagnoses. Patients are often transferred between specialists, as no one seems able to resolve the numerous symptoms, much less find the true source. These patients, with multifaceted symptoms, are often referred to as "List of Symptoms" patients.

Physicians become frustrated by "List of Symptoms" patients, particularly in an insurance-based healthcare system of declining reimbursement. The patients' conditions require considerable effort on the part of the clinician. The current medical system and the seven-minute office visit only lend themselves to looking at a small number of symptoms individually. Thus, many are passed over or passed on to another clinician, often in the psychiatric field.

This 'rejection' by a trusted figure results in a deepening sense of isolation and frustration for the patient. And, it lends itself to a general distrust for the medical professionals. This constant rejection and trivializing of the patient's symptoms can also lead to Post Traumatic Stress Disorder as well. This topic will be covered more in depth later in this book.

Through a patient's journey to find an appropriate diagnosis, they usually start with their Primary Care Physician. The internist can be viewed sometimes as the gatekeeper, since it is often the PCP who must issue referrals to specialists. Sometimes the PCP will write a prescription or two, or send the patient to the next level for evaluation.

Since the 1970s, the number of physicians practicing as general internists has been continually dropping. The "money" in medicine, thanks to the insurance industry, lies in "specialized medicine." Thus, more physicians have become specialists with ever-narrowing focus on revenue – generating activity both in and out of clinical research settings.

Dr. Mozayeni shared a medical school newspaper cartoon that goes roughly like this..." when you graduate from medical school, you know a little about a lot of things. Then, as you progress through your internship and residency and then specialize, you learn more and more about less and less until finally, you know a whole lot about very little."

Specialists are important in medicine. But their specialties have become so refined and restricted, it is often very difficult for the physician to look at the "big picture" and see the patient as an entire "system." They tend to look at the one part and not the whole, repeating their learned rote skills and techniques on as many patients as justifiable.

Even within the world of specialists, many have been trained in medical school to simply address the symptoms; not necessarily to find the source and resolve what is causing the symptoms. If your knees hurt, here are some painkillers. If your blood pressure is high, here are some pills. If you have diarrhea, eat more fiber.

Physicians seem to look more for the diagnosis code to be used in billing and less for the root cause. And thus, they do not cure; they simply mask.

We must ask our physicians to start looking again for causation; not only to give us something to mask the symptoms.

If we do find ourselves lucky enough to find a "Lyme specialist," there are still many physicians out there who will treat "Lyme" disease only. They do not test for or treat co-infections of Lyme. And often the LLMDs do not consider a full range of non-infectious causes of the condition or consider other treatments than antibiotics. Thus, regardless of the approach or philosophy, there are problems with any less-than-capable process of evaluation and treatment.

Patient-Physician Relationship

I think the healing really does not begin until the trust is there within the patient-physician relationship.

When trust is not present, there is

resistance to suggestion and to treatment.

I had one patient who, every time I presented my theory about why she might be sick other than Lyme Disease, she was very polite but became noticeably uncomfortable. She leaned away from me and rolled her eyes slightly.

In a very polite way, I finally looked at her and I said, "I have a feeling you really do not want to consider any other possibility about why you might be sick. I am not dismissing your Lyme. I am simply telling you there might be simpler explanations that you need to explore; that we need to cover. I feel like you do not want to have a conversation, because every time I mention anything other than Lyme, you roll your eyes. I see that look on your face and know you really do not want to consider it."

I had to be very direct with her. I happened to have in the room with me a nurse practitioner knowledgeable in regards to mind-body and the emotional aspects of things and she looked at the patient and said, "Are you afraid? Is there something you are afraid of? Let's talk about it."

And that opened her up and she said, "Yeah I'm afraid."

"Well, what is it? How does that manifest?"

"At night I can't sleep unless there is someone lying next to me. Sometimes I have a friend come over and lie down next to me because I can't fall asleep".

She is a single mom. She is worried about losing her job. She has four children ranging from 9 to 18. There is a lot of fear and anxiety and vulnerability, and she doesn't have another person in her life to protect her and make things okay. So she had this big fear. "If I stop antibiotics I'm going to get sick," she said.

I replied, "You've had a lot of treatment, though, and your inflammation markers are fine. You have nothing on your blood smear and yet you have this metabolic problem that we need to look at. You are a little bit better because of the treatment you've already had, so I want to work with you – but you have to have an open mind about all of these other possibilities."

Establishing and maintaining trust is important. We know some patients have post-traumatic stress from the medical system before they arrive. One of the first things we do, even during the new-patient screening, is to put the message out there: "Look, we understand you, we know what this is like. We know what you have been through and we actually need to talk to you about it directly because unless we move past that, you are going to bring it into this next doctor-patient relationship and we then cannot have true healing." It is a whole post-traumatic phenomenon.

This is key. Our system has trained so many people to not trust. How does one heal without trust? You cannot. The patient must somehow learn to overcome these intrinsic insecurities; physicians must understand their resistance and help them overcome it. This can be a powerful, transformational journey for both.

SHARON

The anxiety I walked in with to Dr. Mozayeni's office with was almost suffocating. I had spent decades trying to figure out what was wrong and how to heal. I didn't know if he could help me or not. There were a lot of questions, a lot of doubt, and a lot of fear. I still had to wait six months before I felt an inkling of hope that I actually might be able to get better. I didn't dare use the word, "heal," yet. At least I thought he might be onto something. But I had to trust him. That was a big step for me, as I think it is for many patients.

DR. MOZAYENI

For a physician who is very empathetic towards patients and wants to help them, it drives you absolutely crazy when a patient thinks you may not be predisposed to treating them for Lyme as *Borrelia* only – when in fact you could not be more sympathetic and capable.

But again, it's the trust factor – that and education. At least most of us have heard of Lyme. But when a physician starts bringing in words like *Bartonella, Babesia, Ehrlichiosis*... it gets lost in translation, and it creates a gap. It took Dr. Mozayeni two hours of explanation and education to get me to buy into the *Bartonella* diagnosis.

During treatment, too, the patient doesn't always see the healing occurring. It can take a long time. This is when the trust in the physician comes into play. Even when I plateaued I never stopped trusting. I believed. I think this was key. Even when Dr. Mozayeni wasn't sure what to do next I knew he would eventually figure it out.

The LLMD has a lot of work to accomplish in each appointment.

Psychological Characteristics

From my experience, I have found most of my chronically ill friends to have the following similar characteristics. They are:

- Anxiety
- Cognitive impairment with significant auditory processing difficulties
- Chronic fatigue
- Feeling out of control of their lives and their bodies
- Constantly trying to "read up" and educate themselves on anything relating to Lyme Disease in an effort to feel a greater sense of control over their disease.

- Sense of isolation and loneliness
- Sense of guilt
- Depressed
- Willingness to try almost anything / Desperation
- Determined

Let's look at these one by one.

Anxiety

I believe the anxiety is produced by the bacteria; directly or indirectly. It relates back to the small vessel disease and neuro-inflammation. Anxiety is caused in part by causing mild cognitive impairment and executive dysfunction. And now we know the brain has a lymphatic system and it is connected to the deeper cervical lymph nodes.

When I finished my *Bartonella* treatment, I was amazed by the significant amount of anxiety that had completely disappeared from my world. Yes, I still experience anxiety, but nothing to the degree it was a few years ago. Dr. Mozayeni kept reassuring me the anxiety was part of the disease, not a bi-product. I didn't really believe him until I saw it actually leave my daily thought process. I had grown up as a worrier (which makes me even more convinced that I contracted *Bartonella* or some other infection at a very young age); anxiety was a very familiar feeling to me. To have it leave my thought process was a little strange, but oh so welcome. Hang in there. It really will resolve itself as you heal.

Cognitive impairment, with significant auditory processing difficulties

I thought I was stupid, not very bright. There were days when I sat in front of my computer screen and did nothing. I could not sort the papers on my desk. I could not pay a bill. I could not answer the telephone. I could not read a book. I could not track the action of a television program or movie. I could not keep track in a recipe to cook dinner. I could not map out how to get to a new place (this was in the olden days before standard GPS or smart phones with directional aids). I could not remember appointments. I could not remember the four things I needed to get at the grocery store. I could not remember to put gas in the car.

We had a saying in my house: "If it doesn't get written down, it never happened." Jeff would verbally remind me to bill a client. But if he didn't put it in writing, send me an email reminder, or add it to my calendar, it did not get done. I could not remember simple tasks, and I could not process what he was saying to me.

At some point, he was certain I was forgetting his items at the grocery store on purpose. But if I went there for three things I needed and he added three more, it was three too many for me to remember.

Chronic Fatigue

We all seem to have different symptoms, but the most common I have found is the fatigue. This isn't the type of tired where you take a nap and feel so much better. This is fatigue that sometimes doesn't lift for years. Yes, years.

It's a tiredness that kept me from sitting up in a chair for more than a few hours at a time. It's a tiredness that makes me lie down flat in my bed, my head level with my heart, almost every single day.

It is fatigue at a cellular level - so deep, so impenetrable, I felt as though I might be sucked into the earth's core.

I still experience this fatigue more often than I want to admit. But I also know now that rest is an *essential* part to healing. If my body is saying it is tired, I MUST sleep more, lie down longer, run fewer and shorter errands. I MUST reduce my emotional stress. I MUST not try to "keep up." It is the only way to heal.

Feeling out of control of their lives and their bodies

When this overbearing fatigue and these migrating, roaming, bizarre symptoms strike, it is easy to feel a loss of control. We canceled countless dinner and lunch dates. We didn't go out much, period. I could never count on my body being strong enough to participate in daily activities. I never knew when it would say, "We are done for the day." When you don't know these things, it creates a sense of fear, frustration, and anxiety.

Constantly trying to "read up" and educate themselves on anything relating to Lyme Disease in an effort to feel a greater sense of control over their disease

This characteristic is an outcrop of the disease. I found myself reading anything and everything I could. But because of my cognitive processing deficiencies, I read a lot of things multiple times and it still didn't sink in. I felt if I understood the disease better, I might be able to control it a little more easily.

While I still try to learn more about this disease, I don't focus on it like I used to. Now, I find it more worthwhile to connect to fellow patients, to share my experience with them, thus ending my sense of isolation.

I leave it to Dr. Mozayeni to worry about the data knowledge research "stuff." He has the M.D. behind his name, not me. I have to trust he is doing what is best for me. I remember in 2009, saying, "Time will tell." It did, and I am so much better.

Sense of isolation and loneliness

Again, because we cannot trust our bodies and brains, we have fewer connections with family and friends. We aren't keeping abreast of the latest happenings. We don't go to movies or watch as much TV or read many books. A definitive sense of isolation and loneliness creeps in.

Certain people close to me didn't really believe I was sick. They thought I had a very low pain threshold or they wondered if I was a hypochondriac (I was actually wondering the same thing).

Finding other Lyme patients who were experiencing similar symptoms was a lifesaver for me. This connection provided me with validation I sorely needed. I was not crazy. I was ill from very real bacteria.

Sense of Guilt

I felt guilty when I could not work a full day. I could not grocery shop. The movie theaters were too loud. The malls were overwhelming. Target and Costco hurt my feet and ankles. A shower left me lying in bed for twenty minutes from exhaustion. Laundry was impossible because my knees couldn't take a single flight of stairs. I got lost driving to places I had been traveling to for a decade.

I forgot to send birthday cards. I forgot to pay the bills. I forgot to shop for birthday gifts. I forgot friends' birthdays. I forgot doctors' appointments.

I wasn't pulling my weight as a human being and everyone around me knew it. It was very humbling. And it was very discouraging.

Depressed

All of the above can obviously lead to depression. Most chronically ill patients suffer from some level of depression. But it can lift as the healing sets in.

Depression can also sometimes mask as anger, especially in men. I believe the Lyme "rage" some patients experience is often masked depression. Be willing to address this issue; don't avoid it.

It is important to share with the practitioner when depression presents. If left untreated, it can devastate the healing process.

Willingness to try almost anything / desperation

I had always been a "western medicine" type of patient. After decades of being let down by western medical philosophy, I found myself willing to try almost anything to heal. I am not as strong a proponent for eastern and holistic approaches as some individuals, including many of my friends. I don't have a whole lifetime of experience with it that so many of my friends do.

I do know there are many people out there willing to sell desperately ill patients anything to make a buck and they have no guilt whatsoever selling a product they know simply does not work.

I also know there are incredibly talented practitioners out there who are healing patients in immeasurable ways and with various modalities.

SHARON

For example, itching became one of my primary 'herx' reactions. Itching *everywhere*. Benadryl was candy; it didn't even begin to touch the depth and breadth of this reaction. I was desperate. I have now found a few things that work for me: dry brushing, FAR infrared sauna, Epsom salt baths (be sure to rinse off afterwards), drinking lemon water, and using soaps made with no chemical additives.

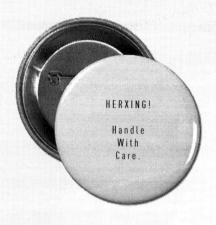

HERXING!

Handle
With
Care.

Definition of Herx

The Jarisch-Herxheimer reaction is a short-term (from days to a few weeks), detoxification reaction in the body. As the body detoxifies, the patient may experience flu-like symptoms including headache, joint and muscle pain, body aches, sore throat, general malaise, sweating, chills, nausea, or other symptoms.

This is a normal reaction that indicates parasites, fungus, viruses, bacteria or other pathogens are being effectively killed off.

The biggest problem related to the Herxheimer reaction is patients stop taking the supplement or medication causing the reaction, and thus discontinue the very treatment that is helping to make them better.

Although the experience may not make you feel good, the Herxheimer Reaction is actually a sign that healing is taking place. The Herxheimer Reaction is an immune system reaction to the toxins (endotoxins) that are released when large amounts of pathogens are being killed off, and the body does not eliminate the toxins quickly enough. This reaction occurs when the body is detoxifying and the released toxins either exacerbate the symptoms being treated or create their own symptoms. Some patients with chronic infections experience mast cell activation when they 'herx'; releasing histamines.

It is important to note that worsening symptoms do NOT indicate failure of the treatment in question; in fact, it is usually exactly the opposite.

The good news about a bonafide herx response is it means the medication is working and your treatment is killing off bacteria. Not everyone experiences Herxheimer responses while undergoing treatment. But if you do, be prepared to experience days when you may feel worse than usual. Pain and fatigue can often accompany a Herxheimer response. They seem to differ for each person.

The pain and fatigue of herxing seems to cycle monthly, usually in correlation with a woman's menses. For men, it runs a bit longer between cycles, about 30 to 35 days.

When a Herxheimer response occurs it is helpful to respond to, rather than ignore, the symptoms. If you are tired, rest. If you are in pain, try heat or detox baths or anything helping to relieve the pain and fatigue. It is important to listen to your body and respond to what you believe it needs.

It might be helpful to write on a calendar that shows the *Month-At-A-Glance*™, this will help give the big picture so when you are stuck in the minutia of "today's a really bad day," you can go back and see that the previous 10 days were great. You know so you're having a better month overall, right now it is the cyclical part that is in the down phase.

Differentiating Between a Herx and a Side Effect

It is important to discern between herxes and side effects.

When you experience a herx, the worsening of symptoms is always followed by a slight improvement in health. That is how you can measure the success.

Some medications will have side effects that can sometimes feel like herx symptoms, but there is no improvement after a few days. I always felt fatigue as a part of my Herx responses, but fatigue was also a side effect of some of my medications.

If you continue to feel a decline in your health over the course of a few months, notify your physician so treatment can be adjusted if necessary. We will cover this topic more in depth later in the book.

Determined

The people I have met over the past four years, all suffering from chronic illness, are some of the most determined, strongest individuals I have ever met. They experience significant pain on a daily basis that they have learned to integrate into their lives because there is no other choice.

- They are determined to educate everyone around them about this disease and the horrible consequences when left untreated.
- They are determined to lead productive lives.
- They are determined to heal in any way, fashion, or form possible.
- They are determined to share their experience, strength, and hope.
- They are determined to connect with one another and support one another in every positive way possible.

All Those Doctors...

When I first saw physicians for my Lyme symptoms, most had a plausible diagnosis for my symptoms and a treatment protocol that worked – at least short term.

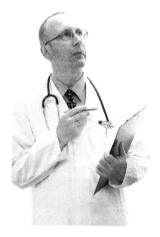

Who is going to argue that hot flashes and irritability are not menopause?

Gallstones? "Female, Fat, and Forty" was the medical mantra for diagnosis. I fit the mantra, therefore, no reason to search any further.

Have a tooth that is dying by itself? Pull the tooth, put in an implant and it's over.

Diarrhea and stomach pain? That's how my body handles stress.

Doesn't every woman have a little incontinence after childbirth?

It all sounded reasonable.

The problem was two-fold, though.

First, no one seemed to be looking for a causative agent. How many patients have a tooth die by itself? No infection, no alien implants. It started dying from the inside out. Wasn't it early for peri-menopause?

Well, yes, but not unrealistic. Gallstones? My mother and sister had them, too; genetics explained that away.

Of all the symptoms I incurred during the progression of this disease, the one that hit the hardest and motivated me the most quickly to resolve was urinary incontinence. Incontinence was not my worst symptom; but it diminished my self-esteem more quickly than any other symptom I experienced. My confidence and courage level directly correlated with whether or not I wet my pants each day.

My first experience of incontinence was after Stephen was born, in 1993.

"Do you know what kegels are?" my ob-gyn asked.

I didn't. But I learned. And I did them. The incontinence was infrequent and mild enough not to warrant any dire action. I only needed an occasional mid-day underwear change and it wasn't enough to have to stop a conversation with a friend or excuse myself in the middle of lunch. It was just enough to be annoying.

In June, 2009, I was lying in bed, resting. I sneezed. My pants were wet. By this point in time, the act of getting out of bed brought me to tears on a daily basis from the back pain. The tears didn't stop this day. Is this what my life was reduced to? Was Jeff going to have to take care of his invalid wife who would eventually need a diaper before age 50?

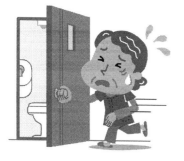 Being wet in my own urine was less tolerable than feeling any amount of pain I had felt to that point. I could handle pain, but I could not tolerate wetting my pants.

One orthopedist, two MRIs, a urologist, and two neurosurgeons later, surgery was suggested to remove a lipoma from the base of my spinal column. Was this the cause of my back pain and incontinence? They weren't really sure. But they weren't sure what else they could do.

Specialists have stopped looking outside their areas of expertise for causes of conditions they treat. There is so much more to learn in each area of medicine. Even to the layperson, it seems almost impossible for medical school students to be able to learn everything even within their specialty.

By the time a physician becomes a specialist, the physician knows a lot within their area of expertise – but many, it seems, are not open to looking outside their particular realm or to look at causes of what lies in their realm. This is probably because so few physicians are trained as medical scientists or researchers. It also seems to me the physicians are not as interested in finding the *cause* of a patient's symptoms. They are quick to address the symptoms, but it seems to be less of an entire disease process evaluation.

"So what's causing the numbness in my hands and feet?" I asked my neurologist.

"We don't know," he replied.

We? Was there a mouse in his pocket?

"What do we do from here?"

"We wait. If the symptoms are still there in a year, we will retest you to see if there is any progression and to see if anything shows up then," he stated flatly. He had already closed my file. Appointment over.

The dentist was fine with taking the tooth out and replacing it with an implant.

"But *why* did it die?" I asked.

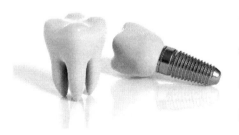

"We don't know," he replied. I guess there was a mouse in his pocket too. "It's some sort of auto-immune response in the body. For reasons we don't know, it will sometimes start attacking itself." His comment propelled me into a vision of a middle aged toothless woman attending her son's high school graduation.

"Does that mean I can lose more teeth?" I asked.

"Not necessarily," he responded. "We don't really know. I've only seen this happen to one other patient in twenty years of practicing."

"I thought you said there was only one other patient who had ever lost a tooth this way. So she lost more teeth?" By now, I was almost pleading, my anxiety level not even remotely hidden.

His silent grimace halted any further discussion. I didn't ask how many teeth she lost.

How Most Physicians Think

Jerome Groopman, M.D., wrote an eye-opening description of medical school training and teaching that fit perfectly into the matrix of why I had so much difficulty reaching an accurate diagnosis from so many physicians. In *How Doctors Think*, Groopman wrote:

"To establish a more organized structure, medical students and residents are being taught to follow preset algorithms and practice guidelines in the form of decision trees. The trunk of the clinical decision tree is a patient's major symptom or major laboratory result, contained within a box. Arrows branch from the first box to other boxes. For example, a common symptom like "sore throat" would begin the algorithm, followed by a series of branches with "yes" or "no" questions about associated symptoms. Is there a fever or not? Are swollen lymph nodes associated with the sore throat? Have other family members suffered from this symptom? Similarly a laboratory test like a throat culture for bacteria would appear farther down the trunk of the tree, with branches based on "yes" or "no" answers to the results of the culture. Ultimately, following the branches to the end should lead to the correct diagnosis and therapy." (p. 5).

But what happens when the symptoms are varied and vague? What happens when the test results are indeterminate? Clinical algorithms work well for strep throat; they do not work so well for vector borne infectious diseases. Algorithms work when the thinking is linear. They do not work when a physician needs to think outside the box and look at the big picture.

Groopman also notes "language is still the bedrock of clinical practice. We tell the doctor what is bothering us, what we feel is different, and then respond to his questions. This dialogue is our first clue to how our doctor thinks." (p. 8). If the doctor is thinking in terms of an algorithm, the questions will be presented in terms of yes and no instead of open-ended queries. This prevents the patient from offering more clues, more hints. Another physician describes the issue as the Tyranny of the Chief Complaint.

Chronic Illness and the Cascading Effect

A chronic illness is not merely a group of symptoms that starts on Day One and continues following a cascade of causation until successful treatment ensues. A chronic illness is a series of layering symptoms unfolding from a chain of events. It is what happens to you after the onset of the original symptom set. The later layers of symptoms are not necessarily based on the original infection; rather they seem to be complications of the original infection. It is a cascade of unfolding events, one leading to more, and progressive decline and destabilization.

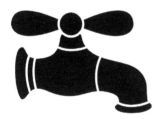

If you have a dripping faucet and you don't know about it for a long time, it might damage the floorboards. There is a sequence of events and if you don't get to it in a long time then your floor beams rot. It keeps getting worse, mold grows and you get mold toxicity. You can replace the floorboards, but if you don't fix the faucet (the source of the problem), or remediate the mold issue, then you will only continue to have problems and more complications.

This is where the "List of Symptoms" patient gets caught up in the vicious cycle. They see specialist after specialist, trying to figure out which symptom came first, which is most important. I had so many issues that were consequences of the original infection, but we never found the original infection until I met Dr. Mozayeni. I knew I had bizarre things happening in my body with no reasonable cause and definitely no resolution. No one seemed interested in symptoms outside of their particular specialty. And certainly no one was interested in finding the root cause of the symptoms. They only prescribed medications to alleviate the symptoms.

TO THE FAMILY
AND FRIENDS

DR. MOZAYENI

As the spouse, significant other, or any family member, **you must be aligned with the patient and, most importantly, you *must believe* this family member is truly ill.**

That is the first step of support. You cannot blame their symptoms on their lack of effort, or see them as someone who is complaining or who is griping.

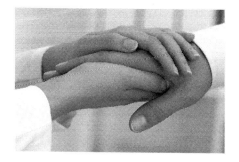

Without medical knowledge and without the experience of dealing personally with the effects of this disease, you cannot proclaim that the only explanation is they are whining or not trying hard enough. You must believe this family member is ill and support their fight.

SHARON

When I shared with friends who also have Lyme Disease that I was writing this chapter, I received an overwhelming response of what they wanted me to include. Of all the chapters in this book, I probably feel the most responsibility in writing this one.

Fatigue

Fatigue is probably the most common characteristic of being

chronically ill. It is the type of weariness that determines what your day holds. Lyme fatigue is unlike anything else I have ever experienced. It is not a matter of feeling tired. It is not the exhaustion at the end of the day.

Lyme fatigue dictates rather than suggests. Lyme fatigue is the tiredness where I come home from work early, at 3 pm, go straight to the bed, push my shoes off and fall asleep within seconds. Sometimes I slept for four hours, awakened for dinner, took my medicine, and fell back asleep until 6 the next morning. Lyme Disease fatigue attacks at a cellular level.

Even as I am healing, fatigue remains my most annoying and limiting symptom. It can take more than hour to get ready for work in the morning because I have to rest after each phase, showering, dressing, drying my hair, eating breakfast, and gathering my things together. I can wake up exhausted. I can be fine for three hours and suddenly have to go to bed for the rest of the day.

Lyme fatigue can make one load of laundry too much for the entire day. Deadlines become meaningless. Executive functioning skills usually worsen when fatigue is present. The worst aspect of this cellular fatigue is that despite rest, despite what little sleep I can get, no more energy is generated. At the deepest levels, my brain and body know no further energy is being created. The fatigue is usually constant, no matter what the patient does; never abating until the end of treatment.

For many, Lyme fatigue is the most lethal component, because along with depression, it removes every chance of fighting.

When I rest, I don't mean sitting on the couch watching TV. Resting means my head is level with my heart. I am lying flat. I often have the lights dimmed, the TV on low if on at all. My senses seem hyper-vigilant when I am fatigued thus necessitating extra peace and quiet.

As I come out of this illness, I seem to have two remaining characteristics:

First, it remains difficult for me to get out of bed in the morning and to get ready for the day. I move more slowly and less deliberately. Maybe it will change, but I seem to be slow to start.

Second, I cannot stay up or out late. By 8 pm, I am ready to get into bed with my pajamas on and lying down. I can be sitting up a bit, but I need to be more horizontal than vertical. I no longer have energy in reserves. I simply cannot do as much as I used to be able to do or attend as many functions as I used to be able to.

Human Being/ Doing

For decades, I believed my value in my community (and family) was directly tied to the amount of work I accomplished. At the day's end, if I had not accomplished whatever amount of work I had subjectively determined as enough, then my value in relationship to other individuals was less than.

When our son Stephen was born with multiple health issues, I found it extremely frustrating at 5 pm to realize the only thing I had accomplished in the day was to take a shower or make the bed. And I still remember one day, when, at 4:45 pm, I had done neither, I rushed into the bedroom and pulled the sheets up so I could state to anyone who might ask that I had indeed at least made the bed.

I did not understand the importance of BEING. I had spent the day (and many others) being a mother, feeding my child, changing him, talking to him, holding him, loving him. That, in and of itself, was enough.

Sixteen years later, in the middle of a herx, I spent the entire weekend lying in my bed with the television on. I didn't take a shower, I didn't get on the computer, and I didn't get up for anything other than the bathroom. Every trip to the bathroom took great concentration, focus and energy. I remember remarking that walking the twenty steps to the toilet felt like a marathon. I'm not exaggerating. My brain and body were so exhausted even breathing seemed a great effort. Jeff brought me food and drink and my pills. I had no physical or emotional energy to do anything. It was an effort to even watch television.

I remember Stephen coming up to spend time with me, lying next to me on the bed as we watched "AstroBoy" on cable TV. I fell asleep for most of it, pretending to stay awake, but my snorts and chortles revealed the truth to the teenager beside me. At the end of the movie, I teared up, apologizing to Stephen for not being able to do anything for him the weekend, further infusing my motherly guilt.

"Mom, don't you get it?" Stephen asked. "I don't need you to DO anything in order for me to want to spend time with you. Lying here watching 'AstroBoy' together is ok. I want to BE with you."

My sixteen year-old boy was ok with simply sitting with his snoring mother. That's when I accepted I could be a human BEING instead of a human DOING. I realized it isn't anything I DO that makes me more or less valuable to others. Rather, it is who I am as a human BEING.

Yes, the things I do for or with someone can flavor a relationship, but they don't change the basic value of the relationship. I didn't need to keep tally anymore of "what have you done for me lately?" I need to be present. And, at a time like this, when even being present is difficult, I can let others be present for me.

The irony was not lost on me that it took a day spent with my baby boy sixteen years later to bring me back to the acceptance that it's ok to spend a day being instead of doing.

But You Have to Work, Right?

For me, I was very lucky to own my own business. I could manage my work hours without a boss hanging over my shoulder. I had a couple of part time employees who could take over for me during the worst days. And I learned to give up on my perfectionism during those rough times. I couldn't do it all.

I know many patients who have lost their jobs, gone into great debt, managing on a one salary income for the family, gone on disability, moved in with family or friends. The horror stories are innumerable, unfortunately.

Some patients have learned new skills that don't require a time clock. Some sell their talents or wares online. I buy many handcrafted items from fellow patients in an effort to support them in any way possible.

I don't have the answer here about how to try to heal and work at the same time. I can only tell you my experience and what I have seen others do.

I had to go back to my daily question: "Will this help me heal?" If I could work, then I went to work. But if I needed to rest, I had to rest. In the end, I realized if I didn't rest, then the work I produced was worthless.

What We Need You, Our Family and Friends, to Know

The rest of the book, I hope, explains the whys of the following list. But somewhere, I think we need to have a list of what we, the chronically ill patients, need you, our family and friends, to hear:

Patients with Lyme Disease or co-infections of Lyme Disease are:

NOT LAZY, FAKING, SENSATIONALIZING, OR IMAGINING THINGS

NOT REFUSING TO LEARN OR GROW, OR AVOIDING RESPONSIBILITY

NOT GOING TO GROW OUT OF IT

NOT CRAZY

NOT CONTAGIOUS— IT IS SAFE TO HUG US

NOT "JUST DEPRESSED"; IF WE ARE DEPRESSED, IT IS BECAUSE OF LIVING WITH LYME, NOT THE OTHER WAY AROUND.

Patients with Lyme Disease or co-infections of Lyme Disease *ARE*:

PHYSICALLY ILL

ACTUALLY, VERY ILL

OVERWHELMED AND FRUSTRATED THEIR BODY CANNOT WORK THE WAY THEY NEED IT TO

EXPERIENCING REAL PAIN, OFTEN EXCRUCIATING

UNIQUE IN THAT WE EACH PRESENT WITH DIFFERENT SYMPTOMS; NO TWO PATIENTS ARE THE SAME

EXAMPLES OF WHAT CAN HAPPEN TO YOUR FRIEND, SISTER, COUSIN OR BOSS WHO HAS BEEN SICK FOR A LONG TIME WITH NO ANSWERS; WE SHARE OUR STORIES SO OTHERS MAY FIND A SHORTER PATH TO A CORRECT DIAGNOSIS

Patients with Lyme Disease or co infoctions of Lyme Disease *DON'T* want to hear:

YOU DON'T LOOK SICK!

ARE YOU EVER GOING TO HEAL FROM THIS? (WOULD YOU ASK A CANCER PATIENT THIS QUESTION?)

BUT YOU SEEMED FINE TEN MINUTES AGO.

BUT I THOUGHT YOU RESTED YESTERDAY.

OH GOOD! NOW YOU ARE BETTER AND YOU CAN GO BACK TO THE WAY YOU USED TO LIVE/WORK!

MAYBE YOU SHOULD SEE A PSYCHIATRIST.

BUT YOU LOOKED FINE YESTERDAY.

I ALREADY TOLD YOU THIS.

GET A GRIP; THERE IS NOTHING WRONG WITH YOU.

SO WHAT, I GET RASHES ALL THE TIME.

IF THIS WAS REAL, THE CDC WOULD DO SOMETHING ABOUT IT.

I KNOW PEOPLE WHO HAVE REAL PROBLEMS.

ARE YOU SURE YOU HAVE A GOOD DOCTOR?

WHEN YOU ARE GOING TO FINALLY BE RID OF THIS THING?

WHAT TIME IS DINNER?

ARE YOU SURE YOU HAVE LYME DISEASE?

HOW CAN ANYONE HAVE THAT MANY SYMPTOMS?

DO YOU REALLY NEED TO TAKE ALL THOSE PILLS?

ISN'T IT TIME YOU GET OVER THIS THING?

Patients with Lyme Disease or co-infections of Lyme Disease *NEED*:

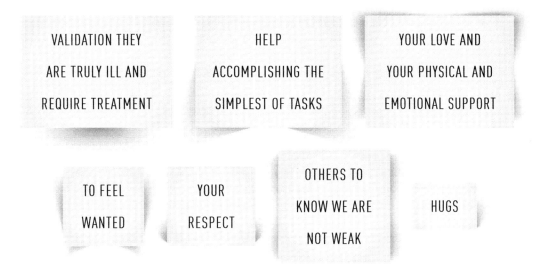

VALIDATION THEY ARE TRULY ILL AND REQUIRE TREATMENT

HELP ACCOMPLISHING THE SIMPLEST OF TASKS

YOUR LOVE AND YOUR PHYSICAL AND EMOTIONAL SUPPORT

TO FEEL WANTED

YOUR RESPECT

OTHERS TO KNOW WE ARE NOT WEAK

HUGS

LOVED ONES TO MAKE AN EFFORT TO EDUCATE YOURSELVES ABOUT OUR DISEASE	ROOM AND TIME TO TO TELL OUR STORIES	FRIENDS AND FAMILY TO LISTEN TO THOSE STORIES
TO BE REMINDED OF THINGS	FUNNY CARDS, FUNNY VIDEOS, OR A NICE NOTE	A RIDE TO THE DOCTOR

Is this Really a Deadly Disease?

SHARON

In 2002, two years after receiving a tick bite, my Aunt Betty died from complications of Lyme Disease. I know others who have died and many more who have *nearly* died from complications from the disease and complications from their treatment protocols.

I also know too many Lyme patients who have taken their own lives as a result of losing all hope for any type of recovery or healing from Lyme Disease. Over the past six years, within Facebook support groups, we lose about one chronically ill patient a month to suicide. While we work hard at staying connected with one another, sending funny or inspirational cards to one another, staying up late with those in crisis, some patients choose to end their own suffering through suicide. This deadly aspect heightens our sense of time; time left in life, time lost to this disease.

This is not a disease to be taken lightly. It is not a disease to ignore. The patients are not faking it or lazy or trying to get out of anything. They are sick and need long term, serious, qualified medical help. They need the genuine love and tangible support of every person around them.

Message from One Caregiver to Another

The following excerpt comes from Sharon Hillje, the wife of a Lyme patient. The question was asked on a social network discussion board, "How will my life change now that my spouse has been diagnosed with Lyme?"

Sharon responded with this:

> Your life is changed. Throw all expectations out of the window. You will need to be three people, at least. Dig in and refuse to be cowed by whatever comes - this is the test of your relationship and your commitment. This is long-term caregiving. This is unconditional love. This is for better or worse, in sickness and in health. And it's the most rewarding and selfless thing you'll ever do. Except it is NOT selfless. Because the bond you are forming with your dependent spouse is greater than most couples will ever know.

You may have to be her hands, her legs, her ears, and her mouth - with chronic Lyme, most likely her brain. She will feel guilt for needing you. You will feel guilt for not being able to make her well. You will need to take some time away for yourself to recharge. It's ok. Love each other and show your children what it truly is about. It is so worth it.

Tips for Family and Friends

Don't ask open-ended questions - give me a choice, but don't leave it open.

When someone asks, "What can I do for you?" Give them a specific task. -Examples - Will you call me on the 15th of each month and remind me to pay the electric bill? "Could you help me figure out how to set up auto payment or auto minimum payments on credit cards so deadlines aren't missed?"

Advise family that time for relationships has to occur when you can, not on the traditional schedules.

Delegate. You have no choice.

If you can't delegate, learn to let it go.

Tell friends you want to be included. One friend sends me photos of events her family has. Not on Facebook; to ME. It sends my heart soaring.

Bring the party to the ill person. Bring a sandwich, soup, and iced tea. And a cupcake with a smiley. And a small terrarium or something requiring little care (our memories fail us).

Send cards for no particular reason. It's nice to send them and to receive them.

Don't tell me to exercise. I am an adult, highly intelligent, and I am ill. My body tells me what I can handle.

Understand and accept my appearance may change. Makeup, hair care, dressing up no longer apply – I can only do what is easiest for myself based on my income, inability to sit for hours, inability to shop.

Offer to do my laundry once a month, help me sort my pills, put bills in a dedicated spot, set up my calendar.

Help with pets; buy a bag of pet food, walk the dog. Lyme patients love and depend on their pets for support.

If I refuse an offer of help, it may be because you offered something I cannot use.

Jeff Rainey

I sat in the marriage counselor's office listening to my wife talk about having no energy, explaining she can't get out of bed in the morning because she is up late into the night unable to sleep. She complained about pain in her feet and legs, her hands and fingers hurt to the point that she couldn't knit or needlepoint anymore...

As she continued I found myself thinking: She has been sick or had health complaints for all but the first two years of our marriage. I am drained from it. I get up every day and go to work, come home and do all the things she can't or won't do because of her "issues." It has taken a toll on our marriage and on me.

I love Sharon, but this seems like it is never ending, one issue after another and tears... I am beginning to disbelieve these never ending issue from migraines to weird pains, stomach issues. Will this ever end?

When the marriage counselor turned to me I asked, "Can I come see you by myself?" She agreed.

In the private session I admitted, "This is a no win for me and I don't know if I can do this anymore. I look at Sharon and feel the wind get sucked from the room. I feel her collapse both physically and spiritually, but I have had enough of this. I have nothing more to give."

I believe marriage is a sacrament – for better or worse, in sickness and in health, all that – but at this point it had taken all my fortitude to stay in this marriage.

The next counseling session was filled with the negative emotions coming out of me like lava from a volcano. I hadn't realized how much bottled up anger and pent up frustration I had.

Sharon's multiple health issues, never wanting to go out, not getting up in the morning, and I'm a morning person - she is not giving me what I need.

I heard myself say I was prepared to leave the marriage, because my world was being reduced on a daily basis. I didn't have a marriage partner. I was a nursemaid and caregiver for someone I thought was an attention-seeking complainer.

The next meeting with the counselor included both Sharon and me.

"We need to figure this out... or to figure out how to part ways with a plan to support our son," I stated flatly.

Sharon was hurt and I was mad as hell. The anger I felt was volcanic and burst from me as I spewed that I was too tired to keep this up. Sharon had been to this doctor and another doctor; each one costing more money and more time away from work – which meant she was unavailable to me and our son. I was very put out by all this.

We had a few more uncomfortable counseling sessions.

Our marriage hung in the balance.

Then a doctor diagnosed Sharon with Lupus. She was, once again, in tears because by this time she was beginning to think she was crazy. Frankly, I was beginning to think so, as well. We talked about this diagnosis and about us. Sharon told me she was willing to work on us but it would take two to make it work. I agreed, but in my mind, it was because she actually had a doctor put in writing that she indeed had Lupus.

This was in July 2009, but soon we found this wasn't the case – she did not have Lupus – and the seesaw resumed.

I had my own health crisis, too. The year before, I was attacked by yellow jackets in the woods behind our house. In the course of trying to escape I stepped into a deep hole and broke my leg in multiple places. The leg was surgically repaired with multiple screws and a titanium plate. They cut me open along my kneecap for 10 inches. I was restricted to bed and a wheelchair, rolling myself out onto my deck and watching the world for 12 weeks. The surgeon warned me if I placed any weight on the leg before the full three months passed I was putting myself at risk for amputation.

I was dependent on others and especially Sharon. It was not a good thing for a person like me, who is always on the go and never sitting still. One day I rolled out onto the deck and was surrounded by mosquitos. I didn't really think much about it. Days later, I had a huge welt-like pimple appear. The doctor gave me antibiotic injections and said I would be fine but they were worried about MRSA.

The recovery from the surgery was long and filled with issues including a deep vein thrombosis (DVT) in my leg and the possibility of death from a Pulmonary Embolism and a general feeling of unwellness continued for a full year.

During this recovery period, the anger I spoke of earlier seemed to well up more often and at the most ridiculous times. Often, I had no memory of why I was mad, but I felt fully justified. This seemed to play well with Sharon's 'illness' and was often a topic at our counseling sessions.

As we continued marriage counseling, Sharon and I talked about our marriage and our commitment to each other as a couple and as parents. We promised to work on and in our marriage; but now we were both struggling health wise.

Then Sharon's uncle, after hearing all her symptoms and health history, told her firmly she had Lyme not Lupus. Sharon's aunt had been misdiagnosed with ALS and ended up dying from complications of Lyme. Her uncle had become a self-taught Lyme expert and swore to help everyone he could. I firmly believe he saved Sharon's life.

She met a neighbor, who was seeing a Lyme Specialist – Dr. Robert Mozayeni. Under his care, our lives began to change. Soon after, I was able to return to work, and Sharon had a diagnosis tying her issues together. Her treatment protocol was one we believed in.

By this time we were working well as partners again and supportive of each other. I was totally dependent on Sharon during the year following my surgery and there was no doubt as to her love for me or mine for her.

But unbeknownst to me this illness had infected all three of us. Not only had Sharon been diagnosed but our son, Stephen, was, too. Now they were both being treated and making progress. In January 2010, I was diagnosed with *Bartonella* and began treatment, as well.

We knew we would need to strongly bond to make it through this horrid illness.

To spouses, partners, significant others I want to say:
It is so tempting to want to give up on each other, to walk away and end it. The fear and feelings of failure can constantly prey on your mind. When an illness becomes a central focus of life, it can be easy to feel you are no longer important to your partner. Or this wasn't the trip you signed up for. I have been there more than once.

Don't give up.

When the going gets tough, go deeper. Reach into your spirit.

We prayed. I prayed. We talked a lot about us and getting through the hell our lives had become. Talk is good.

Accepting that a good relationship is like a marathon, not a sprint, is crucial. The treatment knocked the heck out of Sharon. She was bedridden for days at a time, unable to work, barely able to walk, often lying in bed, eating and going back to sleep.

I had very few problems with the treatment and medications. We did what we could and kept holding each other and talking about what was happening so we could support each other. This went on for 20 months or so. There were lots of up and downs, including some very low lows during those months.

One of the ups – thank goodness for those! – within four months of beginning treatment my anger left me. It was and is completely gone.

Dr. Mozayeni believes I have had *Bartonella* for years, since I too had the multiple hide-and-seek issues that can be part of *Bartonella*, a.k.a '#Lyme Disease':

- heart palpitations
- arthritis issues
- joint issues
- sudden intense pains
- cluster headaches and
- chronic sinus issues

All of these started cycling through my life from about age 24. Back then, I was told I would be in a wheelchair, because I had arthritis in my hip so bad. Then, it disappeared. I'm sure the lengthy infection directly and adversely impacted my life and my relationships over the years.

It is work, hard, daily work, to support and love a spouse, partner or family member with Lyme and co-infections. But it is vital. Every patient needs, wants and deserves to be loved, believed, respected, and cared for.

They are not crazy, or "attention seekers." They are not making this up. Each and every symptom is real. They are in pain. They are confused. They have very real problems making simple decisions; even miniscule day-to-day decisions are difficult.

It is hard to describe the exhaustion because it is so bone and soul deep. The look in the eyes of the infected is deep-set, far away pain and angst ridden. The hurt is at a cellular level. I found often, the only thing that helps is holding them and reassuring them they are loved and that I am here for them.

It is this depth of unconditional love we must wrap them with. Love and compassion are healing.

CASE STUDIES

John (age 53) - Multiple Sclerosis

As a small animal veterinarian, John had daily contact with animals for more than 30 years. Starting in late 2004, he suffered numerous progressive neurological symptoms, debilitating enough that after being a runner for years, he faced the possibility of being wheelchair bound. His hands became numb, and he was constantly fighting fatigue. The buildup of symptoms over months prevented him from maintaining his practice and had him seeking medical help.

John consulted with numerous physicians and was ultimately diagnosed with Multiple (MS), for which there is no identified cause or cure. Physicians began to administer interferon treatment. The treatment may have helped, but John was still concerned. He knew, as a veterinarian, he had been exposed to numerous pathogens, and the MS diagnosis did not explain all of his symptoms.

John tested positive for *Bartonella henselae*. John was placed on a multi-drug oral antibiotic regime that lasted over a year. Progress was not immediate, but over the course of months, John regained significant use of his legs, had dramatically increased energy and saw a reduction of the neurological symptoms. John's quality of life improved to the point he was able to increase his work hours.

Lauren (age 34) - Postural Orthostatic Tachycardia Syndrome (POTS)

Lauren was working as an emergency veterinarian in Washington, DC. In 2004, she received a cat bite during an examination. Within a single day, the bite became infected. Lauren was hospitalized and given IV antibiotics. While in the emergency room, she began to feel dizziness and developed blurred vision. Lauren assumed it was from exhaustion but was still feeling symptoms after three or four days.

Lauren was placed on oral antibiotics and returned to work. During the next few weeks, her symptoms worsened. Her vertigo increased and she grew increasingly tired and weak. She was unable to stand for long periods of time and had to stop performing surgery because her vision was too poor. Her increasing dizziness reached the point that she could no longer drive to work. She also started having trouble focusing and had problems with her short-term memory. Within three months, Laura had to stop working completely.

Lauren saw more than 20 physicians including the Mayo Clinic in 2006 where she was diagnosed with fibromyalgia and dysautonomia, specifically POTS (Postural Orthostatic tachycardia Syndrome). POTS is a chronic illness that is characterized by the body's inability to make the necessary adjustments to counteract gravity when standing up. Patients experience tachycardia (rapid heartbeat), constant headaches, dizziness, weakness, and extreme fatigue.

Essentially, this meant that a single movement like standing up could cause her heart to beat so fast she could pass out. Drug treatments were helping, but Lauren was still very disabled. From 2006-2009, she was essentially wheelchair bound and could not leave her house.

In 2009, after three yeas of POTS treatment and six years of being disabled, Lauren went on antibiotic treatment for over a year and saw slow improvement in her symptoms.

Lauren is now able to drive and go out of the house without assistance. Her energy level is higher and she has regained some independence. She still suffers from blurred vision, some aches and pains, but she is hugely improved today compared to the same point a year ago. She remains optimistic she will be able to resume a normal life. She recently gave birth to her first child and is doing well.

Joseph (age 61) - Asthma and COPD

Joseph is a veterinarian with his own practice in Florida. Before displaying symptoms of *Bartonella* infection, he was an avid bicyclist and enjoyed working on his farm. In 2006, he began to develop severe flu-like symptoms over the course of weeks. These included headaches and fatigue, but escalated into a violent cough. Joseph also began to experience neurological symptoms including tremors in his hands. He had trouble focusing, remembering details and developed short-term memory problems.

After visiting at least eight physicians, Joseph was diagnosed with Asthma and COPD by a pulmonologist. However, those chronic conditions do not typically appear quickly. He was concerned his diagnosis did not fit his condition. Despite treatments for Asthma and COPD, his symptoms were getting worse. He eventually required surgery for sinusitis that developed after experiencing the flu-like symptoms.

Within six weeks of oral antibiotic treatment, Joseph saw improvement. The end of his drug regimen alleviated his cough and sinus problems. Over the next year, his neurological symptoms resolved and he is back to doing many of the things he enjoyed before his symptoms appeared. His memory has returned to normal and Joseph has been able to maintain his veterinary practice.

Hans (age 20) - Hypotension

Hans, a college student in Minnesota, was an active child growing up. He enjoyed hiking, biking, skiing and had pet dogs. He enjoyed a lively social life and was an honor-roll student. In April 2006, the year before high school, Hans began displaying what appeared to be allergies when he broke out in hives and had itchy eyes. However, an allergist was not able to explain the origin of the problem.

These symptoms quickly progressed with the development of insomnia and headaches, followed by light sensitivity and short-term memory loss. His parents were very concerned and consulted numerous physicians, including a neurologist, ophthalmologist, and infectious disease doctor. None of these physicians was able to offer a specific diagnosis, instead only treating symptoms.

After two years, Hans' condition worsened. His energy level was so low he was unable to attend high school instead relied on private tutors and home schooling. Because he was unable to take part in the things he had enjoyed growing up, Hans began to develop anxiety and signs of depression.

Hans had been tested for seemingly everything. He was diagnosed with hypotension and put on medication for his blood pressure, but the only treatment offering significant relief for his symptoms was acupuncture.

Hans found his way to Dr. Mozayeni and started on a long-term antibiotic regimen. At age 20, Hans now enjoys the highest quality of life he has experienced since middle school. He is able to drive and attends college classes. He is able to catch up on the social life he missed out on as a teenager. His energy level, insomnia, headaches, and light sensitivity can still be problematic, but as he continues treatment, he has great optimism.

Brittany (age 21) - Celiac Disease

Brittany, a 21 year-old attending college, arrived at the doctor's office complaining of bloating, gas, and diarrhea.

Brittany had been diagnosed with Celiac disease three years earlier in her home state of Colorado Springs, CO and successfully adhered to a gluten-free diet since then. She also stated she had started to lose more hair than ever before, increased fatigue, and a low grade, unexplainable fever.

The gastroenterologist ordered a colonoscopy and suggested she try a dairy free diet. He also drew blood to check her thyroid. The tests came back all within normal limits. No need to return, he stated.

"But what about my hair falling out? The diarrhea? My fatigue?" Brittany queried.

"We don't know," he replied. "Keep your diet gluten-free and dairy-free and you should see some gradual improvement."

"And the fever?" she asked.

"You probably just had a virus. Make sure you get plenty of rest so your body can fight it off."

Brittany left, frustrated once again.

Brittany's symptoms had not restricted her lifestyle to the degree that things were impossible, but they were a major inconvenience. She didn't go shopping with her mom because she couldn't stand the thought of standing in lines and walking for hours. She chose her outings carefully based on their proximity to a bathroom in case the diarrhea hit. Otherwise, she was a reasonably healthy 21 year-old college girl.

After two hours in Dr. Mozayeni's office, Brittany had a reasonable explanation for every symptom she was experiencing. Blood work results later proved his theory correct.

Bartonella is a chronic infection.

Chronic infection can cause chronic inflammation.

Inflammation worsens the function of the weakest part of a person's body. For Brittany, it was her gut. The chronic inflammation in her gut made her susceptible to allergic reactions. When you introduce grains and dairy products to an inflamed area, you are more likely to produce an allergic, or aggravated response. By omitting those allergens, the response will disappear, but it still doesn't address the cause of the inflammation. Eventually, the bacteria will find another place to attack. In Brittany's case, it was her thyroid and metabolism.

She started to lose her hair. But because she already had thick hair, her symptom was dismissed as insignificant.

"Everybody loses about 1000 hairs each day. You're just becoming more aware of it lately." Even though the thyroid test results were within normal range, the physician didn't acknowledge this symptom was a significant change in Brittany's body and should be addressed as such. And it didn't fit in her category (or his specialty) of the Chief Complaint of diarrhea.

Brittany became lethargic, often worsening when she returned home to Colorado Springs on break. But because she was a college age student, the physician assumed she was not taking as good care of herself as she needed to. And, if he could resolve the Chief Complaint of diarrhea, she would probably develop more energy as a result as well.

Chronic inflammation can make it hard to tolerate high altitudes because the body does not receive as much oxygen as it does at lower altitudes. Less oxygen means less circulation; which means more inflammation. That is why Brittany became more tired when she went home. Her diarrhea increased when she was home. Her gut was more irritated and more likely to respond to any aggravating factor.

While removing the possible irritants from her diet was helpful, it still did not address the underlying cause of Brittany's symptoms. The gastroenterologist felt he had resolved the issue by having her omit gluten and dairy from her diet. Her Chief Complaint has been resolved for most the most part (but not entirely). But the gastroenterologist never looked a layer deeper to find the cause of the inflammation.

Because the other symptoms of low-grade fever, hair loss and fatigue didn't fit into the same category of his specialty, the diarrhea, they didn't fit into the algorithm and thus were discarded as insignificant, irrelevant, or at best, "does not compute."

Axel (age 2) - Chronic Inflammatory Demyelinating Polyneuropathy

When he began to develop rashes in 2009, Axel tested positive for a number of food allergies and was placed on a strict diet. The rashes continued. His mother became concerned when she noticed small bite marks as well as raised blisters. The health issue: young Axel had been bitten by Woodlouse spiders, which huddle under fireplace logs or in warm household crevices.

Over the next 18 months, Axel's symptoms worsened progressively. He had constantly swollen eyes, which were thought to be linked to allergies, as well as low energy levels, chronic sinusitis, and pain in his joints and mouth. Eventually, he developed an extreme sensitivity to light.

When Axel's pain increased at the age of 2, he was diagnosed with chronic inflammatory demyelinating polyneuropathy (CIPD), a rare autoimmune neurological disease. He required intravenous immunoglobulin (IVIG) treatment every four weeks to modulate his immune system. This treatment was difficult and made Axel feel sick, but his physicians believed he would be healthy after six months.

Axel remained on IVIG treatment for more than a year without improvement. His mother took him to see a pediatric chiropractor to help deal with the pain. The chiropractor was the first to suggest the symptoms might be linked to a vector-borne infection and recommended Axel tested for Lyme Disease.

Axel tested positive for *Bartonella* from Galaxy Diagnostics. He started antibiotic treatment under Dr. Mozayeni and the family saw improvement within weeks. His strength and coordination improved, his chronic pain subsided and he was removed from IVIG treatments.

Lynn - Tick Bite

Lynn's journey began during a family football game on Thanksgiving Day, 2006. She pulled a tick off her arm later in afternoon. Two weeks later, Lynn developed a fever and back pain. She had no rash. She thought she had the flu. She mentioned the tick bite to her physician, but he assured her it was too early to see any symptoms of Lyme Disease. Nevertheless, he gave her 28 days of Doxycycline.

She returned a month later, still complaining of vertigo and back pain.

"You are anemic. You need to eat more protein."

One afternoon, during a trip to the shopping mall, she had to lean down and place one hand on the floor and one on the wall to keep the world from spinning. The doctor treated her for an ear infection.

They ran the ELISA test twice, both returned negative.

Two months after her tick bite, Lynn's personality was completely flat. A small group of girlfriends had flown from Texas to surprise her for her birthday. All she wanted to do was sleep. She couldn't understand the jokes her girlfriends were giggling about.

By the end of January, she was in the Emergency Room with such fatigue she couldn't catch her breath. She was jumbling her words, her speech slurred. This 34-year old mother of two toddlers was showing signs of a stroke.

A CT scan revealed peri-carditis. She was sent to a cardiologist, then a neurologist, and an endocrinologist. She visited nationally acclaimed medical centers in the Midwest, Florida and Virginia.

She said they told her they don't know how to treat your Lyme, but we can tell you how to eat differently.

"Become a vegan," one physician suggested.

From January through April, 2007, Lynn didn't drive because of the vertigo and because she had gotten lost while driving the three blocks between her home and her daughter's school. Significant memory loss followed. Her church started bringing dinners over because she was burning dinner every night. "I would forget I was even cooking any food," Shannon admitted.

Two years after her tick bite, Lynn tested positive for *Bartonella* in Dr. Mozayeni's office. Her brain and heart had become inflamed from the chronic infection.

Within months of starting treatment, Lynn was driving, cooking meals, and engaged with her two children. She even celebrated with a "Lynn is Back!" party with friends at a local restaurant.

Laura (age 22) - Bipolar Disorder and Schizophrenia

As a young child, Laura had a number of risk factors for exposure to *Bartonella*. She spent time around animals, her family always had cats, and she spent a great deal of time outdoors. In 2000, Laura's family moved from New York to Raleigh, NC after which she began having neurological problems. Laura was ten years old. Symptoms started with a loss of feeling in her hands and hallucinations. Later, she lost her depth perception and peripheral vision. Over the years, the hearing in her left ear deteriorated and she suffered from chronic headaches.

Laura saw numerous specialists including a neurologist and neuro-ophthalmologist, but all the diagnostic tests they ran to determine the cause of her symptoms were negative. She was eventually diagnosed with bipolar disorder and schizophrenia. Treatment prescribed by her psychiatrist helped reduce her hallucinations, though they were still a problem.

Laura battled with these symptoms all the way through high school. Understandably, school was difficult for her as she dealt with an additional and different set of priorities than the typical teenager.

When Laura started oral antibiotics, she saw small improvements within a few weeks, and feeling returned gradually to her hands – something she had not felt in more than nine years. More results came approximately two months after her treatment ended and included improved vision.

Today, her vision is great, her feeling of touch is back in her hands, and her psychiatric issues are gone. Her physician is weaning her off medication for bipolar disorder and schizophrenia and thus far she has experienced no relapse of symptoms.

At age 22, Laura has a great outlook on her future. She loves her job as a veterinary technician and plans to begin taking prerequisite classes for veterinary college admission.

SECTION FOUR

MATCHING PATIENT, PHYSICIAN & PROCESS

66The good physician treats the disease; the great physician treats the patient who has the disease.99

– SIR WILLIAM OSLER,
CANADIAN PHYSICIAN AND
FIRST CHIEF OF MEDICINE AT THE
JOHNS HOPKINS HOSPITAL

FINDING THE RIGHT PHYSICIAN

The First Appointment

I lied on the 22-page "Complete History Form" Dr. Mozayeni asks all patients to fill out. I suspected if I revealed all of the symptoms I had experienced over the years, he would surely think I needed a psychiatrist rather than an LLMD. No one has that many symptoms without being a hypochondriac; even I had to begun to believe this. I focused on my major symptoms and denied the less compelling ones.

I was very nervous at my first appointment with Dr. Mozayeni. Partially, because I couldn't believe I might actually have Lyme Disease. If I did have Lyme, I didn't want to have Aunt Betty's outcome. And I didn't want to have one more physician looking at my paperwork and giving me another incomplete, inaccurate diagnosis. My anxiety had reached a new peak.

It wasn't like getting a splinter in my finger. I couldn't remember getting the splinter. I couldn't see the splinter. I couldn't get a pair of tweezers to excise it. I knew I felt pain and it kept getting worse. But there was no red, swollen, site with puss coming out. There was nothing to show a physician except my own perception and recording of symptoms. Even some of my lab work was faulty, skewing the puzzle more so. For years, I watched and listened as physicians provided little explanation and less treatment for pain that was increasing sometimes exponentially. Over those years, my anxiety increased, my defensiveness grew.

I talked with other people, researched the Internet (not necessarily the best idea), desperately seeking answers. When I did receive a diagnosis, I thoroughly researched that condition, becoming as expert as a non-science major can become. But when I met new physicians and explained previous conditions, my knowledge base was met with skepticism and obvious discomfort. I found most physicians did not appreciate being challenged by laypeople. I discovered an ugly dimension in medicine.

When the physicians could not come up with a plausible diagnosis or effective treatment, they did not like being put on the spot. They did not care for being challenged with the possibility they might be wrong in their diagnosis. They furrowed their brows, reinforcing their rejection.

In his book *How Doctors Think*, Jerome Groopman points out "physicians, like everyone else, display certain psychological characteristics when they act in the face of uncertainty. There is the overconfident mindset: people convince themselves they are right because they usually are." (p. 150). Groopman adds, "Specialists in particular are known to demonstrate unwarranted clinical certainty.

They have trained for so long they begin too easily to rely on their vast knowledge and overlook the variability in human biology."

Here I was, thinking, **Ok, that diagnosis wasn't right, so what else could it be?** I was ready; no, by that time, I was *desperate* for another possible diagnosis. But the physician was still stuck on the fact that I had informed him he was wrong. He did not like it one bit. Instead of saying, "Let's move on to the next round of possibilities," he suggested *counseling*. I received this suggestion from more than one physician.

My frustration compounded with each visit. I had to *prepare* and brace myself for each physician, to explain why I knew so much about various conditions. I had to emphasize the three most exasperating symptoms to have them even acknowledged. I only had about 11 minutes for each visit and I wanted as little of the time spent in a defensive mode as possible. The urgency and stridor in my voice increased.

I eventually wondered if my desperation for an accurate diagnosis was presenting as Munchausen syndrome – a type of mental illness in which a person repeatedly acts as if he or she has a physical disorder when, in truth, they don't have the symptoms. They act this way because of an inner need to be seen as ill or injured. They are even willing to undergo painful or risky tests and operations in order to get the sympathy and special attention given to people who are truly ill. I definitely did not want to be seen as a candidate for Munchausen.

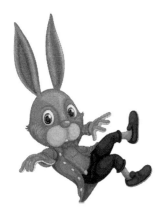

I didn't have an open wound or broken bone. I had migrating pain, tenderness. I had overwhelming, incapacitating fatigue. My hands and feet were numb and cold. I would simply fall. I couldn't walk down the hallway in a straight line. My husband jokingly called me "Ricochet Rabbit." My knees buckled for no known reason. I cried in the morning from excruciating back pain when I tried to get out of bed.

Here was the truth:

I had an inner need to be seen as ill:

first, because I *was* ill and,

second, because no one was validating it

in proportion to the amount of pain I was experiencing.

I had been willing to undergo painful tests in order to find an answer. I wanted my pain to stop. I was willing to go to any lengths to get resolution.

I remember seeing numerous specialists, giving them my thick file, showing them my spreadsheet of multiple diagnoses, many of which were autoimmune disorder related. No one put the pieces together. No one was reading the entire spreadsheet; no one until Dr. Mozayeni.

From the moment I arrived at his office I experienced something different from my other doctors' appointments. I approached the private sign-in sheet sitting on an open counter. There was no sliding window for the receptionist to separate herself. I signed in and sat down in spacious chairs lining the walls against the deep blue painted walls. This room was rich in color, warm, comforting.

Abstract paintings added texture and depth, offering each person their own interpretation to the finished product. There was no right or wrong in this room.

When my appointment time arrived, Dr. Mozayeni came out to the waiting room greeting me warmly with an extended handshake and a genuine smile continuing past the introductions. He escorted me down the hall to his office, one corner filled with diplomas, fellowship certifications and class photos. I wondered which young student was him. Minus the white coats, it could have come from my own college era. We were not far apart in age.

His desk was sparse, more blank forms than ones filled out. In fact, the only file on his desk was mine. No distractions except the telephone and his MacBook laptop.

He opened the conversation by mentioning he had read through my file but he wanted to review my symptoms in a more thorough manner (more thorough than the 22 pages I had answered?).

Dr. Mozayeni went through the symptom checklist and blood work results very slowly, meticulously, often re-asking questions about the symptoms. I didn't have the checklist in front of me, and I couldn't remember which questions I had answered truthfully and which ones I had 'minimized.' About half way through, as he went through each section, developing his theory for diagnosis, Dr. Mozayeni started to explain the *Bartonella* disease process and how my seemingly unrelated symptoms fit together.

Dr. Mozayeni's expression remained open throughout the two-hour appointment. This was a very different experience. His face indicated no judgment, surprise, or condoning. He made direct eye contact with me; his tone of voice was interested, calm, searching, and genuine. He asked open-ended questions. His word choice indicated compassion, humility and understanding. His voice remained calm and clear. As time passed, my anxiety lessened. I would not have to be defensive or demanding in this appointment. I could simply tell my story and relay my observations and symptoms and let him process it from there.

"I have to assume the patient is telling me the truth," Dr. Mozayeni later explained to me. "I have no reason to suspect the patient is lying to me. I have to take the data they give me and figure out how it fits into the system."

Mainly, I was impressed by the amount of time Dr. Mozayeni spent with me, the depth of information he gathered, and the clear intention with which he listened – *really* listened – to me.

From our very first meeting, I have been fascinated watching him. I have learned from him the way he views patients.

Each patient presents like a slide puzzle, a series of square tiles within a border, with one piece missing so the squares can be moved around but in a particular order; more intricate than a Rubic cube. Based on the patient's symptom history and test results, Dr. Mozayeni moves the pieces around within the square until he can finally see the larger picture that illuminates once each puzzle piece

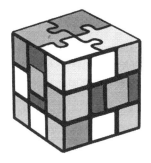 is in its correct place. But in this slide puzzle, because the body is a series of systems working together, the individual puzzle pieces also change shape as they sit within the larger square. It's a combination of a jigsaw puzzle, slide puzzle, and Rubic cube.

Dr. Mozayeni is a fix-it guy. He wants to understand how the body works in order the treat the problem.

He doesn't want to treat only the symptoms;

he wants to treat the <u>cause</u> of the symptoms.

He wants to fix patients, not just make them feel better. He cannot stand the thought of people suffering when the problem is not fixed.

Because I already had some results from IGeneX revealing five positive bands, Dr. Mozayeni was able to start me on some medications immediately. He also changed my thyroid medication dosages and added vitamin supplements

"I think with these changes, you will soon find yourself feeling about 20 percent better than you have been," he suggested.

He also ordered more blood work.

This first appointment was tremendously emotional for me. It was the first time in more than a decade I believed a physician was fully attentive; listening, collecting and evaluating data, and presenting a diagnosis that actually fit.

During my first visit, Dr. Mozayeni clearly (and thankfully, slowly) explained 22 pages and almost three decades of symptoms in a clear, concise, believable manner outlining the likely root cause of persistent symptoms in Lyme Disease and *Bartonella*.

He explained simply and clearly what had been happening to my body for almost thirty years; how each system was affected and had complicated the next set of symptoms that appeared.

To finally enter an office where there was no time limit, no judgment, no disbelief, and no arrogance; well, it was simply overwhelming.

When I left Dr. Mozayeni's office two and a half hours later, I sat in my car and wept. I wasn't crying because I found out I had the same disease that had killed my Aunt Betty years before. I cried because I was overcome with the most profound sense of relief I had experienced in recent memory; and the most amazing sense of honest, authentic acceptance. I no longer needed to 'prepare for battle.' I could be forthright and be believed. I could question and not be reprimanded. I could doubt and be reassured.

During my time with Dr. Mozayeni, and with my other physician encounters, I have learned no one will fight for my health more than I will. I have to know my numbers, know my meds, know what to ask, what to say, what to let go and what to demand. It took me decades to find the right physician. It was worth every step.

I have always appreciated that Dr. Mozayeni tells me up front how and what he is thinking. There is no sugar coating. He is brave enough to admit he doesn't have all the answers right now, but he also emphatically states he will keep searching until he finds them. And he does. I don't want a doctor who placates me with false promises. I need a medical professional who is up front with patients and looks beyond the superficial for answers.

While every patient is different and responds to treatment uniquely, I believe the path to healing will usually occur only through the knowledge and talent of seeing a Lyme Literate Medical Doctor who follows the patient-centered treatment principles of the International Lyme And Associated Diseases Society (ILADS). Other patients have used Naturopaths, Herbalists, and even Infectious Disease specialists. But for the sake of this book, we are focusing on the importance of finding an LLMD who can bridge the lay (#Lyme Disease) definition and medical science definition of Lyme Disease. Regardless of their training, I believe the physician must have the above qualities I mentioned about Dr. Mozayeni in order for the relationship and healing process to be successful.

Honesty Between Physician and Patient

Often, unfortunately, I have to point out what I see the medical system has done to a patient.

Patients are often traumatized by the medical system. When you have a chronic condition, you can develop a form of post-traumatic stress from all of those experiences within and around the health care system.

Patients need to realize the importance and critical value of their participation in the healing process. I tell my patients I may have all the right reasons for the way we need to treat them, and I may be completely right about a treatment, but if they are simply not ready, it will backfire. The opposite of a placebo effect will occur.

There is a shared responsibility in healing. I think many patients are not used to hearing that. I believe it is a critical aspect of honesty to keep patients apprised of where we are in their treatment.

Sometimes, for instance, I'm frustrated and don't know what to try next. (Sometimes I also have to explain the frustration: "Look I'm really irritated now but it's not you specifically, it's what this issue represents in the practice.")

I also insist on honesty from my patients.

The physician's job is to manage the patient's underlying symptoms while also developing an effective treatment protocol for the underlying chronic infection. But all this can only be successful when the patient is honest, direct, compliant, and an active participant in the process.

WHAT TO LOOK FOR
IN AN LLMD

What I Initially Looked For

What I was looking for originally and what I would look for or ask for now are a little different. When I started this long journey with Lyme Disease I had no idea the depth of controversy or the variation of treatment protocols. I remember being shocked I had to "apply" to become a patient of these physicians. The whole thing seemed rather outrageous to me.

Now I have been "in the game" since 2009. Now I understand why physicians choose their patients as much as patients choose their physicians. The most important thing a patient needs to do is find a physician who has a similar vision for treatment. If you are not in alignment, the protocol is not going to work and you will have wasted your time and money and precious energy. Often times, the patient is so ill, they may not know what they need or want in a physician. That is why some physicians "screen" their patients. They want to have a successful outcome as much as the patient does.

When I initially met Dr. Mozayeni, I had no idea what his treatment protocol was. I didn't know about PICC lines, I didn't know about herbals, supplements; nothing. At that point, what I wanted was what most patients need. I wanted someone who:

- validates my symptoms and assures me it isn't in my head
- has a good bedside manner; a good listener, empathic, lets me speak;
- has produced results; has patients who are actually healing;
- is willing to be my partner in forming my treatment plan; allowing me to be an active participant in the process;
- takes the time and effort to figure out why previous treatment failed and what my underlying issues are;
- is knowledgeable and on the cutting edge of research and new protocols;
- is progressive;
- is direct, but compassionate;
- doesn't set false expectations;
- takes his time in the appointment; doesn't make me feel rushed;
- looks directly into my eyes when I'm talking
- actively listens.

Now I know more, so when trying to suggest a physician for other Lyme patients I ask them things like:

- Are you willing to take antibiotics?
- How far are you willing to travel?
- Do you feel you must have a PICC line?

I was willing to take oral antibiotics, but I was not willing to get a PICC line. I was willing to take supplements and herbals, though I had very little experience with them and really knew nothing about their significance or impact on treatment.

The Questions I Should Have Asked

Since 2009, treatment for this disease has changed and research has evolved. Testing has improved significantly. Now, if I was interviewing for a new physician, I would also ask:

- Do you test for co-infections? If so, which labs do you use?
- How long does your average treatment protocol last? (none of them like this question)
- What is your philosophy concerning antibiotic treatment?
- Do you prefer PICC lines or oral antibiotics? Why?
- Do you treat other conditions such as thyroid and adrenal issues? Or do you focus on only *Borrelia* and co-infections?
- How often do you see patients? Some physicians set monthly appointments, others every six weeks.
- How do I contact the office when I have a problem that cannot wait until the next appointment or if I have an emergency? What is the best way to communicate with office staff and with you between appointments (if needed)?
- Have you ever tried complementary therapies for your own well being (i.e., acupuncture, energy healing, supplements, cranial-sacral therapy, massage)?

The most important elements of the relationship with your LLMD need to be honesty and trust.

You must be 100 percent honest with your LLMD and you must trust them enough to comply with the treatment protocol or it simply will not work.

There were definitely times during my treatment when I didn't want to do something. How your LLMD responds to situations like this is key. At one point, I didn't want to start a tough phase of treatment because it was a busy time of year for me and I knew the fatigue it would cause. I was in angst. When I went in for the appointment and Dr. Mozayeni recognized the anxiety, he immediately said, "We won't have you start it until you are ready. If we start it any earlier than that, then it won't work. So let's figure out when you think you will be ready and plan accordingly."

That, to me, is a good physician, LLMD or not.

These physicians who treat Lyme don't just repair your body; they repair your soul.

FINANCES

One of the unexpected trials of healing from this disease is the amount of money needed to get through treatment. Money unfortunately can be the deciding factor of whether patients can heal. If they don't have the money, they cannot afford the wisdom and guidance from a trained physician. And without the trained physician, they will only be able to try bits and pieces of treatment. Unfortunately, in order to heal, a patient needs a long, thorough, consistent treatment protocol.

Choosing Your Health Plan

SHARON

Most LLMDs do not participate with insurance plans. It is up to the patient to seek reimbursement from their respective plans. Most patients have had more success in getting some of their treatment covered when they have a Major Medical plan rather than Comprehensive.

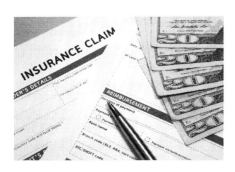

With a Major Medical plan, there is usually a large deductible up front. This allows the patient to choose how to spend the deductible and to make a conscious effort to use it towards the LLMD expenses.

With a Comprehensive plan, much of the choice is removed from the patient's realm. Thus, if they go outside the network, there is little to no reimbursement.

It is also important here to become educated about what conditions the insurance company will and will not approve or cover. Depending on the diagnosis, the physician is usually willing to include a code covered by insurance (as long as it is actually a condition the patient has). This will help ease the reimbursement and approval process.

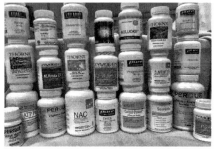

A SAMPLING OF SUPPLEMENTS USED IN TREATING CHRONIC ILLNESS (PHOTO BY SHARON RAINEY)

Most LLMDs will also prescribe supplements, an additional monthly fee. Some will offer these through their practice and others will suggest various places to purchase. It is important to include these supplements in your healing plan. Don't remove them from your daily intake due to cost. They are an essential part of your healing. Figure out a way to budget for the monthly expense when at all possible.

Other complementary aids may help temporarily reduce the symptoms. It is important to remain focused on working with an LLMD to actually kill the buggers and strengthen the immune system simultaneously.

Whom to Treat First?

Often, more than one family member is ill.

Who goes into treatment first? Answer: the sickest one.

As stated elsewhere, this disease can be deadly.

I started treatment in September 2009. Two months later, our then 16 year-old son Stephen developed a sinus infection, then strep throat, and then an ear infection, then bronchitis. We tried four or five antibiotics and he kept getting worse and worse. Finally, the internist tried two shots of Rocephin, which is used to treat bacterial infections... and it worked.

"Test him for Lyme," I stated to the physician.

Stephen's Lyme test was CDC-positive. His *Bartonella* anti-body titers were among the highest Dr. Mozayeni had seen thus far in his practice. Further tests showed Stephen had three strains of *Bartonella* (two of which were the same as mine). We had to initiate treatment immediately.

My treatment protocol was put on hold. Dr. Mozayeni didn't take me off any medications; he merely put me in a hold pattern. We cover elsewhere in this book why it is better when family members don't go through treatment at exactly the same time.

Remember, the sickest or the care-providing family member should be treated first.

Deciding When Not to Treat

Sometimes, families will feel compelled to treat all members even though some individuals may be asymptomatic. If a patient tests positive, they may not necessarily require treatment. If their immune systems are strong and they feel ok, there is no sense in starting the process.

One friend of ours was experiencing fatigue and a general feeling of unwellness. His test results showed 11 bands positive. He was then in the midst of a divorce. He was also an extremely healthy eater, worked out daily and, at age 40, was in the fittest condition of his life.

Dr. Mozayeni suggested some supplements to keep his immune system boosted.

"If you start to feel really horrible at some point," he stated, "Remember that might be the point when you need to be retested and start treatment."

Why would a person who tests positive NOT want to go through treatment? Because the process will usually make a patient feel worse before they feel better. A patient has to be motivated enough to be willing to feel really bad in the short term in order to feel much better, in the long term.

Also keep in mind, however, if that family member is the caregiver for the other sick patients, that task is a stressful burden, which can then compromise the healthiest person's immune system. So be sure to re-evaluate every few months if any changes need to be made.

PREPARING FOR THE MONTHLY APPOINTMENT

SHARON

I start planning for my monthly appointment about three weeks before I go. I know, it sounds crazy doesn't it? But my memory was so poor, I would forget everything over the month I wanted to discuss. When I got around to filling in my Status Update form I couldn't remember anything important. This would result in a wasted appointment and usually more anxiety for the next four weeks.

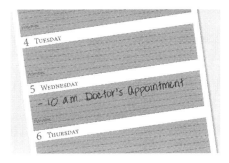

A week after my last appointment, I start filling out my form for the next appointment. I entered the new medication schedule since we decided it a week ago. This is also a good reminder for me to stay aware of any changes I notice in the medication I should alert the physician to.

I add in questions and discussion items, knowing in another week, I may delete them. But this is my place to keep track of what I want to talk about, what my questions are, what I'm worried about.

It's also a good reminder if the physician wants me to get blood work or any other tests done. I get it done that week so I know the results will be in the office at my next appointment.

Under Discussion Items, I would then remember to put in, "Blood-work results."

I also wrote in things like:

- "This medication sucks."
- "How much longer on this drug?"
- "X ray results."
- "I need you to be my cheerleader today and remind me this is going to pass; it's going to get better."
- "My cognitive processing sucks this month. I need your answers

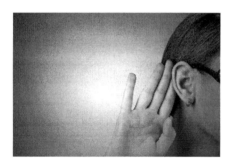

to be one sentence long."

- "I'm tired of coming in here and telling you the lousy stuff. I want to tell you the good things; but I get in here and lose it."

If you have a complicated case, or you know you are about to change things up in your protocol, make your next appointment for early in the week and early in the day, but not on a Monday morning. I know very few physicians who are at their best for a Monday morning or late in the week 4 pm appointment.

If your physician constantly runs late and it drives you batty, then schedule your appointment for first thing in the morning.

The point is: you need to prepare for this monthly meeting. I know it is difficult to do this and for many of us, it is entirely overwhelming in the beginning. But I found when I started preparing three weeks in advance, the final form to hand in was much more comprehensive and clear. It was a useful guide for the meeting.

If you do not prepare in advance, your periodic appointment will be highly inefficient and likely anxiety provoking.

THE
APPOINTMENT

Partners in Healing

Every physician is different; I can only speak to my own experience and what I have heard other patients share with me.

Anxiety is usually a major component in this disease. With anxiety comes some difficulty in cognitive processing. Many patients have found it helpful to bring a friend or family member along for a few reasons:

- It's nice when someone else can drive, thus reducing the anxiety and energy spent in getting to the appointment.
- It's nice to have someone to pass the time with while you are in the waiting room.
- It's nice to have someone else in the appointment to hear what the doctor said, to write it down, to help process it after the appointment is over, to make sure what you think you heard is what was actually said.
- It's a relief to have someone else drive home because you will usually feel physically and emotionally tired.

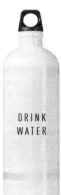

DRINK
WATER

It's also a good idea to bring some snacks with you, (i.e., protein bars, nuts) something to help you keep going. The appointments are usually long and physically draining, so to have a bite to eat can ease the exhaustion. If you bring in fruit snacks or carbs, remember you can have an increase in energy but then a 'crash' afterwards, so something with protein is probably the best idea. A bottle of water is also good to help keep you hydrated. You don't want to bring a whole meal in, or something with a distinctive smell as it can bother other patients. Keep it simple.

Again, the Status Update form and monthly paperwork will usually be your guide for the appointment, so make sure you have your own copy as well as the physician's. Don't count on the physician to go over everything. Make sure s/he doesn't skip anything you need covered! This is your appointment; you are paying for the time.

Come prepared with the information about the details of your health experience during the previous month of treatment. The appointment is for analyzing, making decisions, and being informed about options. It is not about documenting the past month's events – it leaves too little time to review the next steps.

The most important thing to remember during the appointment is your physician is your *partner in healing*.

In order for treatment to be successful, you must be completely honest with your practitioner. If you forgot to take the thyroid meds for three weeks, let him know that when reviewing your symptoms for the past month. If you can't physically tolerate a certain med, let him know this as well. The physician cannot help you if you are not 100% forthright.

One month had been particularly bad for me and I couldn't figure out why. Dr. Mozayeni started going through my medication list. "Did you take 'Treatment B' every day?"

Blindsided.

I had completely forgotten to take the medication. **Knowing honesty and mutual trust is a huge factor in the healing process** I replied sheepishly, I replied, "No, I totally forgot."

"Well, there you go. Titrate back up on it and you should start to feel a difference," he replied.

Through the rest of the appointment, I was silently beating myself up for not remembering.

Finally, Dr. Mozayeni said, "Look, you forgot to take it. It's over and done with. There is nothing you can do to change the past month. It was a bad month and now you know why. So move forward. Start back on it, and we'll see how you feel in a few more weeks." Over and done with.

Forget the shaming, and move on.

(this piece of advice is helpful in

many other aspects of life as well)

That's called teamwork. At the same time, if you disagree with a direction the protocol is taking, you need to speak up. If you don't believe the next phase will work, then it definitely won't. Do not waste your time and energy on something you don't believe in.

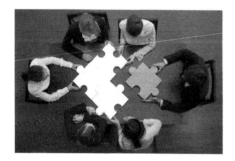

I spent a few sessions with Dr. Mozayeni 'negotiating' my treatment. Not so much in the beginning but more towards the end. In one phase of treatment, I had one particular medication that was working but it made me ill the days when I took it. I was supposed to take it at breakfast and dinner for two days in a row. When I took it, I got a huge immediate herx from it and then about 10 hours later, start to feel better. So taking the second dose was really difficult. After some "discussion," we agreed I would take it three nights in a row and skip the morning dose. He wasn't happy about it, but it was the only way I could manage this particular med at this time.

What I appreciated the most from all this was Dr. Mozayeni's willingness to work *with* me. I know what he wanted; I know what the ideal protocol was. But I couldn't do it.

When Dr. Mozayeni was treating our son, Stephen, he reduced the number of times a day Stephen needed to take medication to just three times a day. He knew a teenager was less likely to follow a protocol requiring taking meds four or more times every day.

It's also ok to tell your physician your emotional needs. There is no one who understands this disease as well as someone else who has it. But your physician is seeing patients all day long with the disease. He understands the process. He knows what tends to happen as you progress through treatment. He gets it. It's ok to tell him about your frustrations and fears.

But also share the good moments with him. They need to hear about the victories as well as the struggles. They need to know what is working for you, not only what isn't working. The positive news keeps the physician motivated; they need the positive feedback as anyone would.

Very Different Priorities & Purposes – The Dichotomous Agenda

When it comes to a patient with chronic illness, the truth is the doctor and the patient have different priorities and purposes for the same appointment. This can be a problem, if not recognized and managed well.

The patient is typically anxious, in a brain fog and suffering from cognitive impairment. They don't know if they're going to survive. They don't know what to do. They don't know what the next day is going to bring. They are in deep need of spiritual healing and spiritual understanding. There is of course the whole mind-body link – so we have the spirit, the mind, and the body. When their body and brain don't work, they are stripped down to their soul.

The doctor's objectives are, of course, to help the patient long-term, but this is complicated by the Western model of the approach to patients - complicated by the rigors of documentation, technical analysis, and technical explanation. While all of this may well be extremely important, it does not meet the psychological and the spiritual needs of the patient. The patient is trying to get those needs satisfied during the appointment and the doctor is trying to be analytical and complete his paperwork so as to keep the malpractice insurers, defense lawyers and the medical Boards happy.

But there is another, deeper issue for the physician, one I had to discover for myself. Whereas in the first appointment I was addressing the emotional needs of the patient I realized in subsequent appointments, instead, I was emphasizing data and analysis. In later appointments, however, addressing emotional needs is as important, because patients don't emotionally heal immediately when you are trying to get them through that physical crisis phase. They are having anxieties and concerns they want addressed, despite the fact you, as their physician, are living in this technical space of the data.

Few doctors who treat Lyme patients want to address the emotional and the spiritual aspect of the patient's well being. They stick to test results and prescription drugs, and protocols or pseudo-protocols. It becomes harder to address the emotional and spiritual aspects after the first appointment because now you have all the data coming in and that consumes more time as it displaces time that would be allocated to emotional needs.

It was stressful to manage an appointment when I knew that while the patient had a therapeutic need for the appointment that even though what I was doing was important, it did not meet the patient's short-term needs to talk through their anxieties, etc.

In my appointments I go through a great deal of data analysis in my head, but I also have to process a great deal of emotionality and constant interruptions with anxiety-driven questions. I gave long detailed answers the patient could not process or remember.

Sometimes this can be an anxiety-provoking experience for patient and physician, which makes the emotionality of the encounter something you want, as a physician, to avoid even more.

The other layer of this is, because I am helping to heal from a place of empathy I start carrying the patient's emotionality. Even though, perhaps I didn't discuss it in the appointment I still feel the emotion. And if I try hard to avoid it I actually make it bigger than it really should be.

Undealt with and carried emotions take a huge toll.

Toward the end of one year I was feeling depressed about what I was doing despite everything positive with many patients I had experienced and what people were telling me. I couldn't quite figure out why. I couldn't put my finger on it. Over the Christmas break I decided to try some energy healing treatment sessions myself.

I was told my heart chakra was badly constricted - so constricted, the energy wasn't coming out of the front of my chest anymore, but out the back. I had effectively closed it off from the front. I was living more in a space of worrying about what was coming at me than taking in what was before me. They say in Energy Medicine to feel it, sense it, but let it pass through. I think I had been feeling it, holding it, worrying about it, not letting it through, and then shutting it out but that became dissonant with my broader purpose and mission.

Most of the patients I see are very empathic, intuitive individuals. I learned I had been getting the very same energy the patients are holding from others, because I was holding from them. Then the energy I was getting from them was the same thing, so I actually was getting it in a recursively severe sort of way and then also doing it myself, much like a microphone – speaker feedback 'squawk' of emotions.

After that experience, three patients came to me, who were in really bad shape. Rather than addressing their issues and symptoms analytically I began to tell them my story with regard to this issue and it tremendously resonated with all three of them.

It occurred to me the way I explained it and my approach to the whole appointment had suddenly changed and that immediately turned my stress into relief.

Normally the appointment would be to review the data and as I did so, I would be pelleted with obsessive anxious questions about what this data means and what that data means these questions were driven not because the patient had a technical ability or desire or need to understand the data. Rather, it was driven by their anxiety to try to grasp and understand where they were in their overall journey as a result of this "milestone" technical information. Truthfully, a technical explanation really doesn't answer that question for a patient.

Tackling the issue head-on and embracing it and making it the center of the conversation and moving all the technical stuff to the side, served to make the appointment easier and more satisfying. The patient left feeling tremendously fulfilled by the interaction instead of leaving feeling confused and anxious and then sending an email with dozens more questions.

The appointment does not have to be dichotomous in priorities. But if I don't address the emotional priorities then I end up carrying it myself for too long. It is educational for my patients to hear briefly about my experience with patients because they might then recognize it in themselves and learn to let it go.

One of the most important things I learned when I was undergoing EMDR and Somatic Experience therapy: whoever is around me, when they throw energy my way, I have to learn not to hang onto it, not absorb it like a sponge. I need to let it to go through. It doesn't minimize whatever the energy is but it doesn't mean I have to hold onto it and it doesn't make me responsible for it. I think it is a key part to healing. I don't have to take on others' issues or energy and I don't have to feel responsible for other people's feelings or situations.

It's quite empowering, but it's eye-opening to think that after you train in technical fields to understand things at a technical level you find yourself doing spiritual, energetic, mind-body work with them.

At the appointment you have to move away from trying to think you need to teach your craft to the patient. You know the technical side but you need to realize they have come to you to heal. That's a pretty big realization because you are talking to them like they are eager medical students who are trying to learn your craft. I kept asking myself, *Why are they asking me technical questions? They have no background to understand the explanations.*

Then I realized their questions are mostly driven by anxiety, generated by the need for control, perspective and emotional support after going through medical encounters that left them traumatized.

SHARON

A friend who also has Lyme was talking with me about *Protozoa*. She wanted to know do we really need to get rid of it or is it okay to hang onto. I told her, "Get rid of the thing! I want it out of me!" "But what if it serves some kind of purpose?"

I replied, "Well, it sure doesn't seem to be serving any purpose to me. As soon as we started getting rid of it, I started feeling better." "I don't think I'm ready to let go of it," she whispered.

DR. MOZAYENI

That's pretty profound because it's a pattern she is familiar with.

SHARON

If you are willing to hang onto something that could be killing you because it is familiar…

DR. MOZAYENI

Change is one of the most stressful things in anyone's existence. We even see patients' anxiety levels flaring after they know they are well, wondering whether or not they are going to relapse, and if the choices they make might put them in jeopardy of relapsing again.

An anxiety flare can accompany the completion of treatment, primarily regarding change. The familiar existence of having this disease is now over. During the illness, the patient can feel a certain comfort because people's expectations have been re-set and 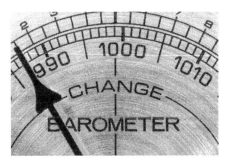 lowered. Now, as the healing happens, you are going to go back to being someone from whom people have higher expectations - and that creates stress. Any change is stressful.

SHARON

I am still trying to find my healthy balance. When I told someone I thought I would probably be healed of all this sometime in the next year, he responded, "Great! Now you can go back to work the way you used to."

I had to say, "No, I can't do work like I used to. That is part of how I got sick in the first place. I've got to find something different."

DR. MOZAYENI

Most patients are transformed by their respective healing process. They now need to find a whole new way of existing, a new lifestyle... a new livelihood.

SHARON

Which is exciting for me, but I can see why it is intimidating for most people.

DR. MOZAYENI

Yes, because you have newfound abilities and insights. Maybe it is intimidating because they had mixed priorities and they didn't start moving; they didn't grow spiritually. They did in a haphazard way not in a sort of guided, controlled way.

There are things they intuitively know that need to be different but it isn't concrete; it isn't very specific so they don't quite know where to go. It's like agoraphobia, a fear of wide-open places; there are too many options out there, too many ways they could misstep. They don't know they can trust their intuition, and they don't know they evolved to have better intuition and more wisdom.

SHARON

And you don't have to do it all at once.

DR. MOZAYENI

Physicians need to realize as patients deal with major debilitating chronic illness, major spiritual or emotional growth phases can occur. This is mostly true of times in which we are in turmoil.

As physicians, we can help patients by supporting them emotionally and in spirit. Those who have inner strength and resilience, who are diligent and stick with it, they get better. They have grown a lot for and through the experience but I think they need better spiritual guides and coaches to help them understand their growth. Then, they can use their newfound knowledge to figure out what they could do differently or what they could do in a better way. Knowing this, they could sense the energy and let it pass through as opposed to holding it could be the best advice they have ever been given.

Perhaps this is a core piece at the heart of healing:

Purpose.

We can help our patients to deal with spiritual issues, by asking then to explore questions like:

"*Why* do I want to get well?"

"*Who* do I want to be around for?

"*Why* do I want to be around?"

"How do I want to *be*, if I am going to be here for them?"

"What can I do to get myself as well as I can be, in order to be around for them in the best possible way?

It boils down to this:

To get well, many people need to come to this conclusion: "I want to get well because there are people I love who I want to help, people I want to be with."

In order for this to happen,

You must learn to love yourself and

not to do things that are hurtful to you.

I encourage patients to keep asking these questions and coming up with a clearer awareness of the important driving forces of their life... and then coming up with plan for how to move forward.

AFTER THE MONTHLY APPOINTMENT

SHARON

For the first two years, and even sometimes now, I was very emotional after each appointment. It took six months of full treatment before I started believing I might actually, eventually, begin to heal.

After each monthly appointment, I found myself physically and emotionally exhausted. It took me days to recover from the appointment. Regardless of how hard I tried to pay attention in the appointment, I only wrote down about 25 percent of what Dr. Mozayeni said. My cognitive and auditory processing skills were severely impaired. I could not absorb most of what he told me.

What I did know was I trusted him. He made me feel safe. He never gave up on me. He listened to me and responded to my needs. He validated my feelings. And he gave me hope. In every single appointment, he gave me tangible hope.

When you plan your monthly appointment, also plan for *after* your appointment.

Immediately after the appointment, I visited a local coffee shop and enjoyed some tea or an almond biscotti; something to let things sink in before I rushed back home into life's routine.

I planned a couple of rest days. I didn't schedule anything important for those two days afterwards. I rested.

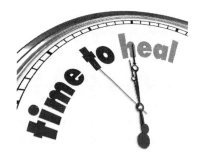

I gave myself permission to feel anything, to process the feelings and emotions connected to the appointment. Sometimes, I would get news in the appointment that took days to sink in. I needed those few days for physical rest, but also for cognitive processing.

After each appointment, I also updated my medication schedule as soon as possible. When I didn't, I would forget at least one medication change he had made, messing up the protocol. I tried to update my form as soon as possible after the appointment.

I wrote a group email to family and friends updating them on the appointment, decisions made, changes in treatment, test results. It was too draining for me to call each person and repeat everything. Writing one group email kept it simple, short, and in writing so I could reference it myself when I later forgot what Dr. Mozayeni and I had talked about.

Be gentle with yourself after the appointment. It is physically and emotionally draining, so give yourself the time and space (literally and figuratively) to rest, recuperate, process, and continue healing.

FRENZIED
FRUSTRATION

There were times throughout my illness and healing when I have felt like giving up. The pain can be too much during a herx. Or I can be in the midst of a really stressful situation. I am usually exhausted. I can't make anything better. I feel horrible physically, mentally, emotionally and physically. It's all too much.

My stress indicators are fatigue, irritability, and light and sound sensitivity. When I am exhausted more than usual, when I am royally annoyed at those closest to me, or when every television, door closing, or dog barking is driving me insane, I know I am in a stressed mode and I need to decompress. I need to find some relief. Rest and quiet are my most significant healers. If I can find a place dark and quiet where I can get my head level with my heart, I can bounce back usually within an hour or two.

Here is what I try, in no particular order:

GO TO BED. I rest, try to nap, keeping the room dark and quiet is often helpful. My body and mind cannot heal without rest. Resting quiets my mind and forces my body to be still.

MEDITATE OR PRAY. I consider these two separate options. I use both, depending on the situation. Sometimes I pray for myself and sometimes I pray for others

DRINK LEMON WATER. It's about detoxing and nourishing my body

USE AN INFRARED SAUNA. Again, detoxing often and being alone in a quiet spot are often healing for me.

GO TO A LOCAL COFFEE SHOP AND WRITE. Writing is my "therapy." Find your therapy and try it.

GO FOR A SHORT WALK. Even ten minutes outside has changed my perspective and/or reduced my stress level.

PLAY WITH MY DOGS. Giving them love, but also playing fetch with them or chasing them in the yard. I have mobility issues, so it's usually fetch. I focus all my time and energy on *them* for a bit.

PET MY ANIMALS.

DO SOMETHING FOR SOMEONE ELSE. Write a note, send a card – get outside of yourself. Let someone else know you are thinking of them, you appreciate them.

KNITTING OR NEEDLEPOINT. I can't do these like I used to because of the pain in my hands. But if you can and you like to it's a good option.

PICK UP THE PHONE AND CONNECT WITH SOMEONE. I rarely do this as I hate using the phone. But others find this comforting and healing when they do it. I am slowing improving at this task.

READ FOR PLEASURE. Nothing academic; read for fun, for escape, for validation, for authenticity.

LISTEN TO MUSIC WITH HEADPHONES.

LIE DOWN AND GO THROUGH THE EXERCISE OF RELAXING EVERY BODY PART – starting at the toes and going all the way up to my head.

TAKE A BATH (WITH EPSOM SALTS IF DESIRED) OR SOAK IN THE HOT TUB IF YOU HAVE ONE. Remember to rinse off afterwards.

DRINK A CUP OF TEA.

PULL WEEDS.

CURL UP IN THE FETAL POSITION AND CRY... OR EXPERIENCE BLISS.

SIT IN A PARK.

WATCH MOVIES WITH A HAPPY ENDING.

CONNECT WITH OTHERS VIA SOCIAL MEDIA. **Remember to "stick with the winners." You want to be interacting with those who are on a healing, positive path.**

EFT TAPPING CAN BE HELPFUL.

PUT ON THE FISHER-WALLACE DEVICE. **(This is covered elsewhere in this book.)**

ENGAGE IN SLOW, DEEP BREATHING.

DO GENTLE YOGA OR SIMPLE STRETCHING.

NETFLIX AND OTHER WEBSITES NOW ALLOW FOR THE INDULGENCE OF BINGE-WATCHING A RECENT TV SERIES... allowing you to soak it all up over a few days with no commercial interruption. For those of us with memory issues this is a luxury.

START PLANNING SOMETHING TO LOOK FORWARD TO when you are feeling better: a mini-vacation, ordering a book from your Wish List, lunch with a friend. (As my friend Linda Hoff said: The exact goal is not as important as having a goal – any goal.)

SURVIVING BETWEEN APPOINTMENTS

Motivation to Change

SHARON

When I received the correct diagnosis I thought treatment would be fairly easy. Tremendously relieved by finally finding the right physician and knowing I was on the right track, I thought it was a matter of sheer will power and determination to get through the next 18 months. I was wrong.

Bartonella is insidious. I was not aware of the comprehensiveness or totality of treatment. It was not a matter of simply taking the prescribed medications at the assigned times. Even that simple task seemed a daunting task at times.

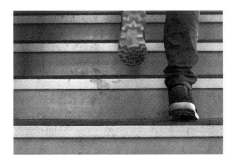

Fortunately, Dr. Mozayeni took me through this process in gradual steps. If he had presented all the changes I would need to make at our first or second meeting, I would have become completely overwhelmed and probably rebellious. I was still rebellious at times with his suggested changes, but every time I incorporated them, I felt better. Feeling better was my primary motivation to change.

It is important for patients to recognize the emotional and cognitive issues essential to managing and mastering the illness.

In almost every lay publication providing advice to individuals about managing their health care patients are told to become as informed as possible and take decision-making into their own hands, because the system can't be trusted to make good decisions for them. This is often true, but there is another important factor to consider.

In these particular cases, because of the level of general debilitation, emotional stress, and cognitive impairment these diseases bring out, it can be difficult for patients to try to understand everything going on. It also makes it very hard for them to actually be their own advocate.

This brings up three major points:

1. *What is the patient's support system, and how do we build on it?*
2. *What can patients do on their own?*
3. *How can the patient have their faith in the healthcare 'system' restored?*

Understanding the Basics

Lyme disease affects all the systems in the body and also impairs mood and cognitive function. It creates a huge emotional stress for the sufferer. The net result is a loss of executive function (organizing and decision-making ability). Because of this, it is important for a patient to understand certain basic things.

For one, if they have limited energy in a day to manage their own care, to do what they need to do, to take the pills and supplements they need, thus spending a lot of their time and energy bandwidth figuring out on their own why they have the symptoms and **_how_** to manage those symptoms will only impede their progress.

It is impossible to look through various websites and social networks related to the available treatment options, to consider all the theories put out there (some of which are not validated in any way whatsoever), to go through all of the data to figure out what is important, what is real, what is relevant, and what is not feasible. To "get more information" is the typical instinct of a sick patient who is desperate for answers. But the core of this behavior lies in the implication:

1. they don't have a practitioner who is competent, or
2. they have one, but they can't trust the practitioner completely because of their own post-traumatic state or traumatic state.

If this is the assumption, the question is: Will _anyone_ be able to hold their trust long enough to help them get well?

Patients' lack of trust in physicians can be a huge issue. When you think about how many doctors are even willing to try and treat Lyme Disease, then narrow it down to the ones who are Lyme literate and adequately treating it, you are talking about a handful of physicians.

Too many people, unfortunately, will not be able to find the individual practitioner with whom they can place their faith and trust. We are not asking people to arbitrarily pick someone and have complete faith in them. That is not realistic.

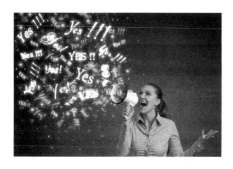

Between appointments, the priorities are to make sure you really know what you need to do and also have constructive ways to manage your emotions and then be careful about how you budget your limited resources of time and energy.

Here are the basics:

- Be willing to try every protocol, if relatively safe.
- Really try it; be compliant.
- Be honest if you have given it a chance and it doesn't work.
- Be honest if it does work.
- Stay focused on the goal of improvement.
- Remember healing can take a long time.

SHARON

Different treatment protocols work for different patients and different physicians match up with different patients; I've learned it is not "one size fits all."

> **Even when patients have the same germ strains and the same physician, treatment protocols may differ according to how the individual patient responds to various medications and modalities.**
>
> **It is imperative we remain respectful of each other's individualized, personalized healing process.**

DR. MOZAYENI

There may be more than one answer to a problem, but the fact is you do much better to follow the protocols suggested by one practitioner at a time.

And once you get into the start of the treatment, you can't continue with the same kind of social network of people who feel lost and negative, and keep repeating the mantra: "I don't know if I am ever going to get well?"

SHARON

Between the appointments it's easy to get into this mindset, especially when you are herxing*

---

* THE JARISCH-HERXHEIMER REACTION IS A SHORT-TERM (FROM DAYS TO A FEW WEEKS) DETOXIFICATION REACTION IN THE BODY. AS THE BODY DETOXIFIES, THE PATIENT MAY EXPERIENCE FLU-LIKE SYMPTOMS INCLUDING HEADACHE, JOINT AND MUSCLE PAIN, BODY ACHES, SORE THROAT, GENERAL MALAISE, SWEATING, CHILLS, NAUSEA OR OTHER SYMPTOMS. THIS IS A NORMAL REACTION INDICATING THAT PARASITES, FUNGUS, VIRUSES, BACTERIA OR OTHER PATHOGENS ARE BEING EFFECTIVELY KILLED OFF.

SHARON

When you are in the middle of the herx, you don't know if it is a herx or if you are getting worse. You don't know until it is over, but by then, the emotional damage is done.

DR. MOZAYENI

Your disease biology itself has a cycle. In between the good parts of the cycle, you have to deal with the bad parts of the cycle. The bad parts of the cycle can make it feel very dark and gloomy. You are deep in a ditch and you can't look up over the edges to see what is out there. This is going to happen more than a few times in treatment. This is when you read the notes you left to yourself to be read on such days.

And avoid negative influences.

I suggest you literally leave yourself messages for when you are going to be in this place. During your monthly appointment or shortly after, write yourself notes saying, "Hey, I've analyzed this plan, I'm comfortable with it. I've got good reasons for doing it, and I'm going to try it for a while. My time frame is about this long and I need to be able to read this note when I'm feeling really down and realize how I was thinking at a time when my mind was clearer and better informed."

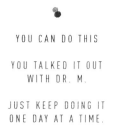

YOU CAN DO THIS

YOU TALKED IT OUT
WITH DR. M.

JUST KEEP DOING IT
ONE DAY AT A TIME.

I think this can help people get through these very low points because they might only trust their own note to themselves rather than conversations with lots of different people.

I also made an Excel spreadsheet to record the dates and tasks I could accomplish again that I could not do the month or year before. I still remember writing down when I could make the bed in the morning again - a significant task for me.

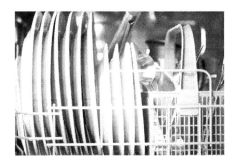

I remember being able to unload the whole dishwasher instead of half. It is a small task, but for me it was big. When I started feeling down and frustrated by what I couldn't do I could go back and look at the list and say, "Well, you couldn't do these things either, but now you can."

It was a tangible reminder I had the energy to do the whole dishwasher or to take a shower and wash my hair or to take less than an hour to get dressed for work. It's the small things but when you are looking incrementally it was big.

You have to remind yourself of where you were then to see where you are now.

I love that, too. Keep a running list of milestones at which you realize you actually can do certain things you couldn't do before. In the early phases of treatment practitioners, close family and friends often see major improvements in the patients but the patients actually don't see it.

We always ask the patients, "What's improved since you started?" and they will often forget, but when we start going back through the "problems list," they are reminded. It goes like this:

- "Oh what happened? – What about this symptom?"
- "Well, that's gone."
- "And what about this one?"
- "That's gone, too."
- "How about this one?"
- "That's gone."

This awareness may not trigger a better mood, but you can clearly see they have improved and the patients actually, literally, have to be shown this. If you are a patient, you can help yourself a lot by keeping a simple list of major milestones of improvement.

Again, it takes patience on the part of the physician, who may keep hearing, "I'm not getting any better." And it takes patience on the part of the patient. If a patient is on a general trend of improvement, the practitioner may need to remind them when they are sick, their frame of reference, in terms of looking forward and backward is very narrow.

The patient may say, "I don't recall feeling better a month ago." They may remember very little in their short-term memory and perspective because of limited executive function, cognitive ability and the stress and strain of the disease. They actually don't really remember how they were feeling very far back in time. As they get better, their perspective broadens. When patients begin healing they don't have a recollection of where they used to be.

The only way to really know it and track it is to be organized about keeping a list. This is an example of where one should spend their time and energy. It doesn't take long to do.

Sit down and ask what you were able to do today that you couldn't before.

SHARON

Sometimes there will be nothing, but other times there will be. It doesn't have to be done every day. Even weekly will do.

It can even be the message to yourself. Instead of feeling guilty about resting all day if it was not a good day, the fact you know you need to rest is still changing your frame of mind and not looking at the list of things not done as something to leave you guilt-ridden. Rest is a hugely important part of healing and it is what you are "actively doing" to heal.

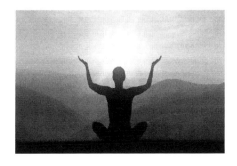

If you don't physically do something on a particular day, you can feel comfortable you at least spent the day meditating and thinking and praying about your healing. Meditating, thinking and praying about your healing is necessary, because healing your body can be a way of planning the next few steps.

SHARON

Even now, these many years later, I still have occasional days where my body says, "You're done for the day." I recently had a weekend where I slept hard for 9-10 hours, and the next day I took a three-hour nap. I had plans for doing something else, but I had to remember what my body needed for the next stage of healing. It doesn't happen as often as it used to, but it happens, and I still need to listen to my body and what it needs for continued healing.

DR. MOZAYENI

And because you rested, you will actually have the energy to do something when your body is ready.

Stay focused on the trends. Do not worry about moment-to-moment or day-to-day changes. There will be fluctuation over periods of days and weeks, at a time. STAY FOCUSED ON THE TRENDS.

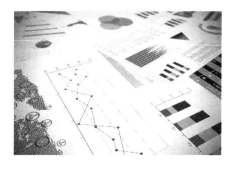

Any journey has bumps in the road and turbulence in flight. If you don't have any, it means you are going nowhere. There are shifts, and with shifts, come stressors. Sometimes the shifts make you a little more uncomfortable for a while before you get better.

Shifts and stressors can occur during a Jarisch-Herxheimer reaction - temporarily feeling worse when you successfully start treating an infection. This is when it is important to leave notes to yourself to chart how your symptoms are changing and how you are improving. Blind faith is then not required.

But you do need to:

have enough faith to commit to a process long enough and to commit to working on a solution with whomever you have chosen to work with.

Communicate to the practitioner your concerns or ambivalences because even though the treatment may be right, if you are not ready for it, it will have the opposite of a placebo effect, called the nocebo effect.

PLACEBO NOCEBO

You must be ready and receptive to the treatment. You need have to a sufficient amount of conversation with whoever is taking care of you to be able to reach the point so you can have confidence to proceed for at least six to nine months with any chosen form of treatment.

Do things to help avoid feeling like you are lost.

This includes the things we have already discussed as well as having a positive supportive network that is helpful to you while you are in the phase.

Be careful not to get pulled into the negative energy of social forums attended by people who have either failed treatment or have not started treatment and are looking for a way to get treated.

Listing for yourself your priorities every day is another important task. Once a day one journal what you did, what new milestones you reached. Keep a prioritized list of tasks.

SHARON

You told me for the first two years the most important priority every day was to put my healing above and beyond everything else.

For every task, the question needed to be,

"Will this help me heal?"
With this one question, it became very easy
to determine what I should do every day.

This entire chapter is interesting to me because each topic it is still all about positive energy.

Every single day, your first priority must be healing.

Everything has to go from there. Whether or not you go to the grocery store – if you can physically manage it – depends on if you can do it, if you are in the healing aspect.

I remember I had to take my son, Stephen, to the grocery store with me for the first year, because I couldn't be in there more than 45 minutes. I'd hit 40 minutes and I'd have to leave my cart, because I couldn't stand up any longer. Planning is all based on what I am going to do to make sure I'm still healing today. I can't go to the grocery store for an hour if I know it's not going to work. Instead maybe I get half of what I wanted. It really became such a minute breakdown of tasks to make sure I kept going in the right direction.

I think many patients have trouble breaking the tasks down, because for many of us it's all or nothing; we don't see how to break it down into manageable pieces; like doing one load of laundry instead of three loads. It becomes that small.

DR. MOZAYENI

If a practitioner is to demonstrate they are trustworthy, they should know all the rungs of the ladder that the patient must climb, as they improve. The patient's job is to climb one rung at a time.

**The practitioner holds the vision of
what is possible for the patient.**

In that sense, the practitioner holds the ladder for the patient. The patient climbs.

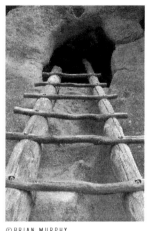
©BRIAN MURPHY

Being positive is absolutely huge. The analogy would be planning a really nice vacation. You need to be thinking about what it is going to be like when you are well and until you can envision that, until you can envision your destination, until you can envision actually being on the vacation you actually won't ever get there. You will never plan for it, you'll never buy your tickets; you'll never actually go there. Some people call this the "Law of Attraction." I call it planning and follow through.

SHARON

I can even see trying to plan what my life would look like once I'm healed, to set this as a goal. But what I thought it looked like in 2009 and what I want now are very different pictures.

I remember Dr. Mozayeni saying to me early in treatment, "You cannot go back to the life you had because it is what got you here. You have to make some big changes or you are going to be right back in the same spot."

The first time I heard this, it was really hard. Obviously as I healed, I realized he was 100 percent right. Trying to communicate this message to people around me was a little more difficult. It was a challenge.

But it is what saved me. To be able to go out during the week at night used to be a big deal. Now, staying home is actually a gift – I don't even want to go out. It is more of a gift when I have time with my family. It is a vision that changed for me as a result of healing.

DR. MOZAYENI

If you had known then it would kind of work itself out then it wouldn't have been so hard.

Sometimes what you think of as a disappointment actually ends up being the gift.

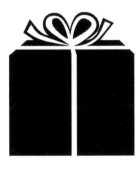

It might be so much better than the routine you had before; something that would not have been possible without this growth phase, a growth period, associated with the lessons from the illness.

SHARON

I read a quote today, **"When you think things are falling apart they may be actually falling into place."**

DR. MOZAYENI

It's analogous to the chronic illness experience patients have. They often find themselves ultimately in a much better place. When one is tapped out of energy, resources and cognition, it may be hard to appreciate, but on a limited basis if they weren't trained, professional healers to begin with, the patients become healers in the course of learning how to heal.

They learn the skills and we think if they help someone who may be a few steps behind them even just a little bit, it could be a very positive thing for them (as long as it doesn't drain their energy). People who are not professional healers often have trouble with the boundaries that need to be set.

SHARON

It's a good reminder of how far you have come. If you are in a group with people who are a little further along in healing and people who aren't quite as far along it gives you a nice sense of where you were, where you want to be, and the possibilities.

DR. MOZAYENI

I have seen, ultimately, patients' lives can be greatly enriched by the experience. It's not one you would ever voluntarily sign up for. Doing this professionally is something only a few would voluntarily sign up for. Like the patients, you find yourself in it if you are inclined by your compassion to solve problems.

Temporary Damage, Not Permanent

Mostly, I want to remind patients and physicians: most of our patients don't have any permanent damage.

And for patients especially, here is the last bit of advice about how you survive between appointments.

Any good day you have is proof that your systems can work normally – it is a 'systems check' green light.

260   LYME SAVVY | TREATMENT INSIGHTS FOR LYME PATIENTS AND PRACTITIONERS

Any hour you have where you are functioning and things are working is proof your damage is not permanent. This is a very, very profound and important point to remember.

I think it is important in your log or journal to keep track, even if you had only minutes or an hour or so of normal function. It is a huge reminder to yourself that your systems <u>can</u> work and <u>do</u> work and it is a matter of time before you are going to get it all there more consistently.

SHARON

It is also important not to sweat the small stuff. Patients can freak out with the peripheral neuropathy, as it comes and goes. Now I can remember it is going to come back. It went away for a little while, but the feeling is going to come back. I have to hang in there and be patient. It's not that big of a deal; it will get there.

DR. MOZAYENI

Using the electrical grid energy analogy to describe this, small-vessel disease is like having small brown-outs throughout a city, but a brown-out in a hospital will have a different effect on a city than a brown-out in a school which is going to have a different effect than a brown-out in a switch controlling the county's traffic lights

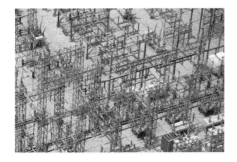

which would have a different effect than a brown-out at the water treatment plant or in a communication cable or sensor. You have these little brown-outs occurring in different spots throughout your body.

Symptoms will fluctuate and they will be in almost every organ or tissue. What freaks out patients is the extent and variety of the symptoms and the fact that they fluctuate. While every symptom can make a patient very anxious, to me it all points back toward a systemic body-wide small-vessel disease process. To me, it can be an affirmation of the fact we are on the right track. It is the thing I have to explain the most often.

SHARON

It seems for the chronically ill patient, things initially are black-and-white. A symptom gets better and you think great, *Done with that, move on* – and then it comes back and you think, *Oh I'm not getting better, I'm not healing*. It's hard for us to see the gray area.

DR. MOZAYENI

There is interesting research establishing that a little bit of chaotic fluctuation actually may stabilize biological systems. For example, an athlete has an intrinsically variable heart rate as do dogs because they have the capacity for high physical exertion. Once a heart rate becomes very steady, it means it's actually responding to some stressor that takes away this inherent irregularity. There is a lot of systems-theory science around how you stabilize chaotic systems but when you have a level of a disease process with system compensation you have a certain level of homeostasis, a certain level of steadiness. When we try to move people from one state of stability to another state, a preferred state of stability, you create some instability on the way to getting there. It's easy to say; it's really tough to go through as a patient.

It is like traveling. You really can't go from point A to point B without encountering some bumps in the road, some turbulence and a little discomfort. To travel, you've got to use some fuel and you're going to spend some money. Typically, when patients are not doing anything and they have a level of illness, they have a certain amount of fluctuation of symptoms where they don't get too good and they don't get too bad.

Once you start treating something, we find you will have days on which you are considerably better than your baseline and you will have some days where you are considerably worse than your baseline. You now have cycling where there is greater amplitude. There is a broader cycling, from better points of improvement to worse points of feeling bad. Gradually, you have fewer bad days and you have more good days but you still have good and bad days.

The trend, as it becomes positive, is not
a straight line, but a cycle with a trend!
Pay attention and focus on the trend!

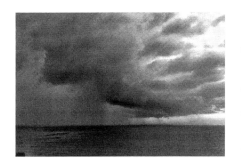

It's a cycle as you continue to improve. When the sky is clearing after a storm, it doesn't instantly go from being terrible to instantly being perfect. Initially, there are fewer clouds, the sun starts intermittently breaking through, the temperature gradually changes, the precipitation may be off and on but it is more off than on as the storm clears. It is important to recognize it is never instantaneous. It is gradual and it is cyclical. You have more and more better days. If you can track the number of good hours in a day and the number of good days in a month you will often see your trend is improving.

As I tell patients, "It is a ride, and every ride has movement and some bumps."

SHARON

Most of the words coming up today, like the **compensation, chaos, fluctuate, shift, cyclical; it's all about trying to get that balance.** We are simply trying to find the balance.

DR. MOZAYENI

And trying to find balance means you are going to be slightly off balance as you are trying to find the new balance.

SHARON

And it's not necessarily a bad thing. When we are chronically ill, we have been sick for so long, we don't know much about balance. It can be terrifying to take one step back when I forget I've taken three steps forward.

DR. MOZAYENI

I think so much of the healing process is about remembering where you are in the overall process.

You have to maintain perspective.

HERXING

SHARON

Definition of Herx

Earlier in the book, we covered the definition of a herx. I want to cover it a bit more in depth here as I know this issue can feel paramount for patients currently in treatment.

To review, the Jarisch-Herxheimer ("herx") reaction is a short-term (from days to a few weeks) detoxification reaction in the body. As the body detoxifies, it is not uncommon to experience flu-like symptoms including headache, joint and muscle pain, body aches, sore throat, general malaise, sweating, chills, nausea or other symptoms.

This is a normal reaction that indicates parasites, fungus, viruses, bacteria or other pathogens are being effectively killed off.

One big issues associated with the Herxheimer reaction is that people stop taking the supplement or medication causing the reaction, and thus discontinue the very treatment that is helping to make them better.

Although the experience may not make you feel particularly good, the Herxheimer Reaction is actually a sign healing is beginning to take place. The classic Herxheimer Reaction is an immune system reaction to the toxins (endotoxins) released when large amounts of pathogens are being killed off, and the body does not eliminate the toxins quickly enough. This reaction occurs when the body is detoxifying and the released toxins either exacerbate the symptoms being treated or create their own symptoms.

It is important to note temporary worsening of symptoms does NOT indicate failure of the treatment in question; in fact, it is usually the opposite as long as it is temporary and followed by a period of improvement. The good news about a bonafide herx response is it means the medication is working and your treatment is killing off bacteria.

Not everyone experiences Herxheimer responses while undergoing treatment. But if you do, be prepared to experience days when you may feel worse than usual. Pain and fatigue can often accompany a Herxheimer response. They seem to differ for each person.

Our son, Stephen, primarily experienced extreme fatigue. Jeff had migrating joint pain and a temporary worsening of his skin rash. My herxes were usually a couple of days spent in bed with fatigue and a temporarily worsened back and hip pain.

One herx included severe scalp and head acne. I resented having worse acne at age 47 than I had at 17. The pimples multiplied daily. They were larger than typical, also tender, painful, red, and gross.

As abruptly as the acne started, it stopped two months later.

The pain and fatigue of herxing seems to cycle monthly, usually in correlation with a woman's menses. For men, it runs a bit longer between cycles, about 30 to 35 days.

When a Herxheimer response occurs it is helpful to respond to, rather than ignore, the symptoms.

If you are tired, rest. If you are in pain, try heat or detox baths or anything to relieve the pain and fatigue.

It is important to listen to your body and respond to what you believe it needs.

It might be helpful to write on a calendar that shows the *Month-At-A-Glance*™; it will help give the big picture so when you are stuck in the minutia of today's a really bad day, you can go back and see that the previous 10 days were great. You know so you're having a better month, right now it's the cyclical part currently in the down phase.

Differentiating Between a Herx and a Side Effect

It is important to discern between herxes and side effects. When you experience a herx, the worsening of symptoms is always followed by a slight improvement in health. This is how you can measure the success.

Some medications will have side effects that can sometimes feel like herx symptoms, but there is no improvement after a few days. I always felt fatigue as a part of my Herx responses, but fatigue was also a side effect of some of my medications.

If you continue to feel a decline in your health over the course of a few months, notify your physician so treatment can be adjusted if necessary.

DETOXING

Importance of Detoxing

During treatment, patients can suffer from a Herxheimer or "herx" reaction. It is also often referred to as a healing crisis, a detox reaction, or die-off syndrome. This reaction is a short-term (from days to a few weeks) inflammatory reaction in the body. These episodes are usually a normal reaction that may indicate parasites, fungus, viruses, bacteria or other pathogens are being effectively killed. Some of the symptoms of a 'herx' may be from a surge of histamine release and depletion of positive mood neuro-transmitters.

Although the experience may not feel good, it is actually a sign healing has started. It is an immune system reaction to the toxins (endotoxins) being released when large amounts of pathogens are being killed off, and the body does not eliminate the inflammatory factors and toxins quickly enough.

General Detox Methods

It is recommended that, if possible, we want to try to help the detoxing process along. Many methods are available and each person responds differently to each type. Below are listed some methods that have worked for patients. The purpose of the detox method is to draw those toxins out of your body in any way possible.

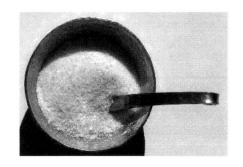

Remember, when drawing toxins out, as with the sauna and Epsom salt baths, you want to rinse off afterward so the toxins are not reabsorbed.

- Infra-red saunas
- Baths using Epsom salts, apple cider vinegar, herbs
- Coffee enemas
- Colonics
- Drinking lemon water
- Drinking tart cherry juice
- Juicing
- Green smoothies
- Apple cider vinegar tea with a spot of honey
- Ionic footbaths
- Various supplements aid in detoxification (ask your LLMD)

Importance of Genomic Assessment in Detox Support

It is important to focus on the individual's tolerance and the processing of the toxins. We can now do a genomic assessment of different pathways of detox in individuals.

As a general rule, patients with chronic symptoms tend to have a higher likelihood of having an underlying host-response problem with methylation, both MTHFR and catecholamine (COMT) methylation. They also seem to have a higher likelihood, particularly if they have neurological symptoms, to have a compromise of their glutathione metabolism and detox functions in their liver. The brain and skin are derived from the neuro ectoderm same tissue embryologically so we find the glutathione transferase is present in one form in the liver (GSTM1) and then two other forms in the brain and skin (GSTP1).

If one is exposed to certain toxins and has a limitation of the glutathione detox function in the liver, then you may be more prone to having neurological and skin problems.

The glutathione metabolism pathway is intricately tied into methylation metabolism. Patients can get sick when you start supporting their methylation because now they are able to process the accumulated toxins and hormones. It must be done carefully, gently and slowly.

It is helpful to look at the detox pathways but I think it is complicated biochemistry and I think it takes a good bit of time for a clinician to develop the skill set to be able to genomically counsel and manage a patient with an impaired ability to detoxify.

Cytochrome Enzyme Limitations

There are many cytochrome enzyme considerations. Cytochrome P450 enzymes in the liver are involved in the metabolism of lots of different drugs and toxins and an individual's genetic profile can tell you a lot about what drugs they can and cannot handle, whether or not they are going to be more sensitive to cytochrome inhibition by grapefruit juice and, for example, whether or not they are slow or fast metabolizers of caffeine.

Any prescription drug given these days should be done with the knowledge of how the drug is going to get metabolized, not in general, but in that individual in particular. One can greatly reduce the side effects and risks if we don't blindly apply the same regimens to every patient. If we can understand them, we can genomically personalize the treatments to minimize the toxicity. Metabolic support, individual pathways, and the careful selection of prescription drugs are all much more important in the whole detox question. The treatment must be precisely personalized to maximize effect and minimize side effects.

Chelation

I have seen patients on chelation protocols who end up getting toxicity from the chelators. Given the long-term implications and outcomes of chelation therapy, a slow and steady approach with sustainable things is best. Chelation of heavy metals is rarely an urgent immediate concern, although it may be important on a long-term basis.

Even Vitamin C in high doses can be a heavy metal chelator. Making sure one's glutathione levels are high can be a very important way to naturally detox and chelate heavy metals. There are some basic things we can do without getting into any kind of crazy chelation protocol where you potentially could make someone sicker.

Don't Make Things Worse

We have all heard of all kinds of therapies and things patients have tried ranging from ionic footbaths to coffee enemas to saunas. Any time you sweat for any reason, you eliminate toxins through the sweat glands. This can be helpful. But sometimes, what you are doing can make things worse. You need to be sure the potential risk, difficulty and cost is somehow justified either in strong patient preference or solid data or at least a reasonable cost and risk benefit analysis that is not just a monetary cost-benefit analysis but also a time-cost-risk-and monetary benefit analysis.

How much time does it take? How much effort does it take? How much risk does it present? These are broad questions, and it has to be personalized down to the level of considering the risk versus benefit and acknowledging the **perception** of risk and benefit is more so the patient's than anyone else's as long as they have good information about the range of options available.

Any nutrient, even water and oxygen, can be toxic if given in excess. "Detoxing" is a general term overused by practitioners and patients who don't really understand who offer various unusual treatments that are perfectly good but given at the wrong time. For some, food sensitivities are the 'toxin.'

When detoxing it is critical to be very clear about what toxin you are trying to address.

You need to be precise about
figuring out what toxin is the problem.

Genetic predispositions can make one person really unable to handle a certain kind of toxin or a medication that another would tolerate well.

It can sometimes be the very simple things you would never consider such as the antibiotic itself. If the antibiotic is not processed properly by an individual given their metabolism, then the very antibiotic that is being used becomes a toxin in the right circumstance. When there are general symptoms that cannot be explained people throw out the word "detox."

"Well, let's detox someone if our treatments aren't working. Let's give them more treatments that don't work because now we have to detox them from the treatment." They use the outcome almost as a rationalization and even for the diagnosis because if the patient is not responding to *Borrelia* antibiotics, the practitioners don't consider that, perhaps, the problem is *Bartonella, Protozoa* or another co-infection. Instead, they invoke the word 'toxin' trying to justify throwing twenty treatments at the patient.

SECTION FIVE

TREATMENT

"I was waiting for the kind of solution where God reaches down and touches you with his magic wand and all of a sudden I would be fixed, like a broken toaster oven. But this was not the way it happened. Instead, I got one angstrom unit better, day by day."

– ANNE LAMOTT, BIRD BY BIRD

MANAGING CHRONIC ILLNESS (FROM THE PHYSICIAN'S PERSPECTIVE)

DR. MOZAYENI

The management of chronic disease differs from acute disease. Acute disease usually has one clear causal explanation. With chronic disease there are usually several layers - several contributing factors. Physicians are taught in training to use Ockham's razor; that there is usually one explanation to explain the set of findings.

With chronic disease I find it is the opposite. There are layers and pieces and you have to look hard and find all of them. You must address each piece. Because you do not know how much each finding contributes to the symptoms, you have to prioritize your approach and not overwhelm the patient with treatments for every single finding. This requires clinical insight, good judgment and an ability to triage all of the potential contributing factors and approaches.

My experience has proven if you do not take a comprehensive, integrative and functional approach, you will likely not have good success rates.

When infections are chronic, if you take a 'germ-only; or 'germ-centric' approach, you will not likely have good success rates.

Clinicians who do not use an integrative approach tend to use more IV antibiotics. They tend to start giving more intense multi-antibiotic regimens, a treatment regime which can potentially make for a very sick patient.

I think this happens a lot. I also believe there are some doctors who have been treating Lyme Disease for a long time, who have not made use of newer, more scientific methods and good logic to diagnose and manage patients with chronic complex symptoms.

Functional Medicine

Functional medicine addresses the underlying causes of disease, using a systems-oriented approach. This approach engages both patient and practitioner in a therapeutic partnership.

Functional medicine is an evolution in the practice of medicine that better addresses the healthcare needs of the 21st century and the specialty training does not teach this approach.

Functional medicine shifts the traditional disease-centered focus of medical practice to a more disease process-centered and patient-centered approach, addressing the whole person, one system and one disease process at a time, not as a set of diagnoses.

Effective functional medicine practitioners spend time with their patients, listening to their histories and looking at the interactions among genetics, environmental factors, and lifestyle factors influencing health and chronic disease.

Functional medicine often integrates traditional Western medical practices with alternative integrative medicine, creating a focus on prevention through nutrition, diet, and exercise; use of the latest laboratory testing and other diagnostic techniques; and prescribed combinations of drugs and/or botanical medicines, supplements, therapeutic diets, detoxification programs, or stress-management techniques.

Some of the most common holistic aspects of functional medicine for chronically ill patients include:

- checking for food allergies,
- genetic metabolic characteristics (methylation and detoxification)
- adrenal function,
- thyroid function,
- mold, and most importantly of all,
- testing and treating chronic infections.

Food Allergies

Food allergies are common in most patients with chronic inflammation. It's a chicken or egg first paradigm. We don't know if it is the cause or the result of a disease process, but it can cause severe symptoms, many associated with inflammatory small vessel disease that can cause neurological problems. I know of a dentist who retired because his hands shook too much. He didn't know he was allergic to gluten. When he stopped gluten years after retirement, his tremor resolved. His daughter was able to stop thyroid medicine after stopping gluten when genetic tests showed gluten sensitivity risk.

None of the current food allergy tests are perfect. The only ones reimbursed by insurance are the IgE antibody tests. Yet many of these food allergies involve different parts of the immune system. The tests are not as good as we would like, but they can be a good place to start. Usually, in severe cases, you can find a very important contributing food allergen. Typically, if the patient then eliminates the food from the diet, the patient will see an improvement in general health.

There are two food categories some doctors will automatically recommend eliminating from a patient's diet even without testing just because the likelihood of a food allergy from these two things is very high. They are **wheat** and **dairy**. After these, the top food allergies are soy and eggs. Grains can expose patients to mold. Other foods can case mast cell activation and histamine release.

Those are the top four food allergens. If you are chronically ill, it is a good idea to avoid these four groups. Soy has the additional risk of being high in pesticides as it is often a GMO food (unless it is organic).

SHARON

I haven't had any major food allergies show up in my testing. But I do know when I keep my diet gluten free, dairy free, egg free and sugar free, I feel A WHOLE LOT BETTER than when I don't. I recently took a trip and ate healthy for the entire week, omitting gluten, dairy, sugar, and eggs. It was a transformational week for me, showing me the power of these ingredients.

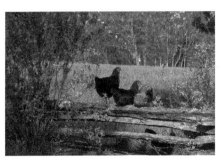

FREE RANGE CHICKENS. DO YOU KNOW WHERE YOUR CHICKENS COME FROM? WE DO! PHOTO BY CRAIG HAGAMAN, HIGH VIEW FARMS, BERRYVILLE, VA

This was much easier said than done and took me more than a year or two of treatment to start some of those changes. I am fortunate in that, upon my diagnosis, my husband started an organic garden in our backyard and now even raises bees so we can eat raw, unfiltered honey.

When I started treatment, I tested high in arsenic on the heavy metal testing. Dr. Mozayeni gave me a report on chicken from 2006 (http://iatp.org/documents/playing-chicken-avoiding-arsenic-in-your-meat). We changed our diet to completely organic chicken and within months, my arsenic levels plummeted.

Some people can make these changes all at once. I could not. I have had to do it in increments.

Methyltetrahydrofolate Reductase (MTHFR) Gene Mutation

The other medical condition that we are seeing in many patients with Lyme Disease co-infections is a genetic deficiency related to the processing of folic acid. It is called the methyltetrahydrofolate reductase (MTHFR) gene. It is responsible for the methylation of folic acid. This form of folic acid bypasses the enzyme and allows the rest of the body to start methylating. It actually supports methylation throughout the body. It is involved in many, many normal processes as well as detoxification pathways. You have to accurately diagnose it and then support it with things that support methylation. Activated folic acid (methylfolate), B12, and other supporting factors such as betaine can help manage this condition.

There is more to the methylation analysis than MTHFR. Some people have an impaired ability to handle sulfur, as in glutathione. Some people who are sensitive to it may also have other methylation issues. Those factors are also involved in methylation. There may also be deficiencies of COMT (Catechol-O-methyltransferase) and this is central to how we process adrenaline and sterol hormones.

When you begin managing a patient's previously blocked methylation pathways, you start clearing a lifetime of processing backlog that has never been done in that person's body before.

You create big shifts. You have to start that process ge...
opinion, in order to minimize side effects.

With chronic inflammation the body holds onto heavy metals more tightly, because, for example, metallothionenes are being produced in excess.

Methylation is important in:

- steroid metabolism,
- adrenaline metabolism (via COMT enzymes),
- detoxification,
- DNA metabolic modulations, and
- DNA imprinting in epigenetic modifications.

That is why this whole process becomes systemic and deep. It is fundamental to our metabolism. It is also potentially very complicated involving many genes and their metabolic pathways.

Mold

Mold issues vary region by region, throughout the country. It can be a significant issue because mold toxins generally activate the immune system. We can still have good success rates without worrying too much about mold but I do think some of the patients have significant mold issues. It can be very difficult and costly to evaluate and manage.

:ity is a whole other area of research and controversy

:he potential to greatly complicate and benefit the care

:nt with Lyme Disease. It is a huge ordeal to deal with any

ne issues that can be affecting a patient, but to also bring

more to the equation adds another dimension. Unfortunately, the testing for and abatement of mold can be very expensive so it is a significant issue that needs more work and attention.

When a mold toxicity problem exists, it can mimic some or all the symptoms of Lyme Disease and/or get in the way of a Lyme patient's improvement.

Adrenal Function

Adrenal function is covered in detail elsewhere in this book, but it is integral to successfully treating chronically ill patients and requires one to look beyond lab tests for symptoms and signs of hypothyroidism as the problem is usually **not** related to the thyroid gland but due to the peripheral (cellular) conversion of T4 to T3 and rT3.

Thyroid Function

Thyroid function is also explained elsewhere in this book. It is an integral part of successfully treating patients.

Testing for Co-Infections

When we talk about *Borrelia,* we must talk about other infections called co-infections. I don't know if there really is anything "co" about these infections. I think they are called co-infections because as Lyme patients' symptoms didn't respond to treatment, people started looking at other infections, especially those other infection that are also maybe carried by ticks.

So which germs really cause Lyme Disease?

Co-infections most commonly found in patients include *Babesia*, *Ehrlichia*, *Anaplasma* infection, *Bartonella* or other proteobacteria, or *Mycoplasma*.

One study done in New Jersey found by PCR, which is not as sensitive as enrichment culture followed by PCR, approximately a third of the ticks carry Borrelia, a third carry Bartonella, 2% carry Ehrlichia and 8% carry Babesia. The positive rate for Bartonella may be even higher if the study were to be repeated using enrichment culture followed by PCR - a method developed later.

Researchers started recognizing the gut of a tick is not a place where the tick only selectively carries *Borrelia*. Ticks, like other insects, can carry various microbes. However, it is not proven that ticks transmit these microbes; and it is not proven that ticks do not transmit them.

It should not take a lot of research to determine this. If a tick is feeding off a variety of mammals why wouldn't the gut of the tick have a whole bunch of different things in it? But it does create some interesting questions. For example, we have never really had a good *Bartonella* test until recently. How can we be really sure the ECM rash or Bell's Palsy are only from *Borrelia*? What if the ECM rash or Bell's Palsy is from both *Borrelia* and *Bartonella*? That is an interesting hypothesis.

Is there some combination of microbe inoculation that has to occur in order for someone to get sick from a germ?

Does it have to be *Protozoa* plus bacteria? Would the same person get as sick if they had only one of those? These are some of the questions related to these infections. The complexity goes up exponentially because now we have to go further than deciding if one of these infections can make someone sick without the others. We need to answer the question, "What happens if a person is dealing with combinations of these germs?" or "What sort of person (genomics, diet, etc.,) would get sick from a germ?"

Broadening the Focus

This leads to a paradigm shift in how we are beginning to think about these germs. We need to start thinking about there being an entire set of genes being carried around by different kinds of microorganisms. We need to think about the whole ecosystem and potentially look at all of the genetic information determining bacterial, microbial and parasitic characteristics. We need to conduct a microbiome analysis of all the genetic material associated with illness and also consider the best response to the genetic code found in that microbiome.

The future of this science will be to look at someone's blood, or even all the parts of their body, and understand the ecosystem of germs living there. You also look at their genome. Then you rent some time on a supercomputer, assuming you know what to tell it to do, to figure out what sort of disease would result, and what the best treatment approach would be for an individual with that genome, this microbiome, this diet, these environmental factors, this sort of stress or this kind of pollution in their environment. When you can run a full simulation considering _everything_, then you know you might be able to get the answer to everything. That is the "pie in the sky."

In the meanwhile, the more comprehensively we look at different germs the more we will learn. We also then need to develop technology to prove whether or not a specific germ causes that symptom.

If you see biofilm in the bloodstream you know it can and will plug up small vessels. You know particles longer than blood cells are not going to flow through arterioles because capillaries let red cells through only in single file. If there is anything bigger than even a clump of red cells it's not going to go through a capillary. Biofilms may even do worse – they may coat the blood vessels and help germs thrive, damage blood vessels, and contribute to or cause arteriosclerotic disease.

We know in the vascular medicine scientific circles
that arteriosclerosis likely results from
long-standing chronic infection localized in a patchwork
in the lining of blood vessels throughout the vascular system.

Given we now recognize this – evidenced by the CRP measure emerging as a better vascular risk marker than LDL cholesterol - we need to understand better the role of chronic infection in the development, progression, and treatment of chronic illness.

Evaluating the Probability for Each

One last point on co-infections: there are greater risks for *Bartonella* as a co-infection of *Borrelia* because you can contract *Bartonella* **also** from flea-bites and cats. Fleas and several other vectors are the risk factors for Bartonella transmission

Bartonella has been shown to be present in:

- fleas,
- dust mites,
- allergen extracts that are used to treat dust allergies by injection,
- bed bugs, and most importantly,
- the common house cat.

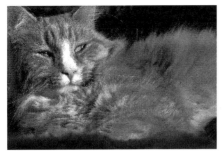
©ANGELE RICE

As I stated earlier, especially if the cat is an indoor/outdoor house cat, it is very likely to be carrying *Bartonella*. The microbe gets into its saliva, the saliva gets onto its fur, its dander and the dander gets into the air. However, currently, there is no evidence to support Bartonella transmission by cats unless the cats are concurrently infested with fleas. When Bartonella bacteremic cats are co-housed with non-bacteremic cats transmission cat to cat does not occur in the absence of fleas. This may or may not be true for dogs - we have no data speaking to this.

Current evidence from cats is that the saliva and nails become contaminated with infectious flea feces when the cat has fleas. While no studies have been done that measure the risks, basic facts suggest a cat owner should be very careful to limit how much time the cat is allowed outdoors in order to reduce its risk for flea and tick exposure. Further, a cat or dog owner should be vigilant about controlling fleas.

**Fleas, including sand fleas, present
a high risk for *Bartonella* infection.**

We try to blame the flea and the bug rather than the pet. Veterinary medicine has worked to develop some excellent products to prevent flea and tick infestations in cats and dogs, which should prevent bartonellosis in family members. The products should be used year round for the life of the pet.

Remember, up to 80% of feral cats may have *Bartonella*. It may be higher. I have found in patients with Lyme Disease a history of much more exposure to cats than to deer ticks. Most cats are completely asymptomatic even when infected. Keep in mind it is when the cat has fleas, that its fleas, scratch or bite is likely to cause Cat-scratch disease and that the cause of that disease, *Bartonella,* is very likely to go systemic and persist after the rash has resolved. This has caused the medical profession to assume that Cat-scratch disease is benign and self-limiting – just because the rash resolves on its own.

No one realizes the rash is only the first phase of *Bartonella* infection and that the commonly involved lymph node swelling is clear evidence of the systemic spread. Once in the lymph nodes, the *Bartonella* causes a form of immune suppression and tolerance thus allowing the disease to appear to resolve when really it is going into remission preparing to cause a chronic smoldering inflammatory process throughout the body.

I think the attention given to *Borrelia* and its connection to the deer tick has gotten far more attention than what is another, possibly higher risk of exposure to fleas and the risk of *Bartonella* infection.

In the groups of patients we have studied, exposure to a cat, or to a cat plus fleas, is a more likely scenario given the prevalence of cats in human households.

Bartonella is a very common co-infection of Lyme Disease.

Bartonella is not just a co-infection of _Borrelia_.

Bartonella can be a chronic infection often unrelated to Lyme Disease.

Bartonella is also a chronic infection often misdiagnosed as Lyme Disease.

And,

Bartonella infection might be a more significant global public health problem than Lyme Disease.

Further, many patients with _Bartonella_ will continue to refer to their condition as "Lyme Disease" in their social networks. I call this #Lyme Disease.

SHARON

I grew up with cats my entire life... how many scratches and bites did I get over all those years? Any one of those could have infected me. I don't recall ever getting a tick bite. It makes much more sense to me that I was infected from one of the many cats I encountered.

Can Bartonella be One of the Biggest Global HEALTH Problems?

All mammals can carry *Bartonella*. It has even been found in whales. Although *Bartonella* has been found in all mammals, all of the attention has been directed to rats, bats and cats.

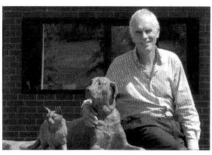

DR. ED BREITSCHWERDT, DVM AT NORTH CAROLINA STATE UNIVERSITY.

Many veterinarians and physicians believe *Bartonella* is a significant global public health microbe. Dr. Edward Breitschwerdt believes that *Bartonella* is a big global **health** problem and at this point in time, it is not fully recognized as such.

Bartonella could turn out to be an important co-factor in some forms of immune suppression, including HIV and Malaria. Some very recent strains of *Bartonella* have been found in AIDS patients. Dr. Barbara Koehler at UCSF discovered a strain of *Bartonella* that was named after her, *Bartonella koehlerae,* in an AIDS patient. Our group published the first eight cases of *Bartonella koehlerae* in immuno-competent patients.

Typically, the medical profession has believed that in human mammals *Bartonella* is only an issue in the immunosuppressed. In our published case series of 296 patients we found evidence of Bartonella in about 62 percent of patients who thought they had chronic Lyme Disease.

Many people with *Bartonella* out there who think they have Lyme Disease, so the term Lyme Disease has become way too broad. It has become the term that the popular, in the vernacular, describes everything that is not understood – it is what I call #Lyme Disease.

Because that thinking – that logic – lives on the Internet, the definition of Lyme Disease keeps expanding. On the other hand, scientists try to keep their definitions pretty tight so they can have logical discussions and move the science forward. They come up with a concept, narrowly define it and give it a name so that they can talk about it and then move it forward.

With the rise of the self-taught citizen scientists and the availability of information on the Internet, there is no logical process to guide a scientific discourse leading to an improved understanding of the problem.

Instead what you get on the Internet and in popular discussion is a flurry of confusion and anxiety mixed with an occasional piece of incredibly valuable information if you can recognize it as you wade through all the blogs of suffering, confused, anxious patients.

Adrenal Fatigue

In a patient with chronic illness, who likely has small-vessel inflammation from persistent infections, hyper-coagulability and poor circulation, there exists also substantial dysfunction and poor interconnection of body functions. In other words, you get less robust interaction among the different tissues of the body including the parts of the brain, the endocrine system and the endocrine system's relationship to the central nervous system.

All of these different functions of the body become disjointed – instead of working in sync, they start working autonomously and asynchronously because of unreliable interconnections and functions.

All of this creates a lot of stress – that stress causes the patient's adrenal glands to run a higher than normal output of the stress hormones, such as cortisol, hydrocortisone, or adrenaline. The adrenals are the main mediator of stress hormones. The outer part produces the cortisol and the inner part produces the adrenaline, the epinephrine and noradrenaline.

In a patient who has been experiencing chronic stress from having highly compromised physical, mental, and emotional function, the adrenal glands will exhaust themselves and use up the substrate as well as the different vitamins and nutrients that go into the production of adrenal hormones. The individual reaches a state of persistent adrenal fatigue.

Adrenal fatigue is a substantial depletion of the adrenal's ability to respond to basic needs and, of course, inevitable environmental stressors. Adrenal fatigue is measured most typically by looking at the diurnal salivary cortisol concentration to gauge actual adrenal function rather than to use a stress test such as the Cortrosyn or ACTH stimulation test.

Symptoms of adrenal fatigue include:

FATIGUE	LIGHT HEADEDNESS	MUSCLE WEAKNESS AND LOW BACK PAIN
BODY ACHES	SLEEP DISTURBANCES	SALT CRAVING
LOW BLOOD PRESSURE	INFLAMMATION	EXCESSIVE THIRST AND HIGH URINE OUTPUT
LOSS OF BODY HAIR		

The traditional view of adrenal function indicates that adrenals do not fatigue; with a little rest, adrenals recover. But remember: chronically ill patients are not able to get enough rest. In addition to all the other problems they have, they can't sleep well. They can't get restorative sleep because their system is fundamentally disordered.

In traditional approaches in medicine, the adrenal is evaluated by stimulating it maximally with the highest possible intensity using the injection of a hormone called ACTH or adrenocorticotropic hormone. An injection of ACTH causes a doubling of the baseline cortisol level over a short period of time of one to two hours. If the result shows the cortisol doubled, then it is considered a healthy adrenal and if it is not, then it is considered a dysfunctional adrenal.

Thus, you have a binary rule where if you meet that threshold, everything is fine; if you don't meet that threshold, the adrenals are not working well or not working at all.

Medicine history unfolds first around the extremes of the diseases, which are the easiest to discover and to describe, and then later medicine evolves its ability to be able to gauge the subtle abnormalities with a more subtle understanding and better tools.

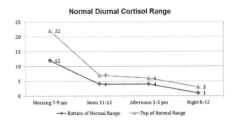

We are at the juncture of appreciating that adrenals are not binary organs. They don't either work perfectly or do not work at all. We have come to understand that the adrenals are organs and are going to have a gradation of function ranging from none to perfect. This is the approach taken by functional medicine practitioners.

In functional medicine, therefore, the saliva cortisol level is used to look at the diurnal variation of cortisol to gauge the level of adrenal function. Patients who have been chronically stressed and have had chronically high production of adrenal hormone will have a depletion of their adrenal output and low or altered saliva cortisol levels. Normally, the pattern would be highest in the morning, and then taper down over the course of the day. Patients with adrenal fatigue can experience low levels in the morning and during the day and then experience higher nighttime levels when their energy finally improves. This is part of the reason they have disordered sleep.

The disordered sleep correlates with insomnia. One of the first things you see with chronic illness is an inversion of the normal cortisol production: lower than normal in the daytime and higher than normal at night.

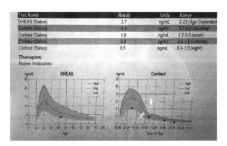

ADRENAL FATIGUE DIAGNOSED IN THIS PATIENT

The patient-reported energy level, in my experiences, correlates strongly with the saliva cortisol level relative to normal. If the salivary cortisol is supposed to be high in the morning (higher than the rest of the day), and it is at the low end of normal for that time of the day, the patient will report fatigue. That lower than normal level at that time of the day could still be a lot higher than it is at night but it all has to do with where the level is relative to where it normally would be determines the person's energy level. At night if the level is typically much lower but then the person has a high normal level (which is still a lot lower than the low normal level experienced in the morning) the patient will actually report higher energy or good energy at night. The patient's measured salivary cortisol level then usually correlates well with their reported energy and their adrenal fatigue with some occasional exceptions.

That's why we can be tired all day long, unable to even get out of bed, and then at 11 pm, it's like someone gave me a sugar and caffeine pill. It drove me crazy. For years, I would cycle with staying up until 4 a.m., then crashing, absolutely unable to wake up when needed later that morning. It was never an issue of will power; it was an issue of the basic adrenal energy was simply not there.

Other times I was able to work all day, then I'd come home and fall on the bed and be asleep within moments, not minutes. I would sleep for three hours solid, wake up, eat dinner, and go back to sleep for another 10 hours.

This was my first sense of having no control over my body. As much as I wanted to do things, my body simply shut down and required me to do nothing but sleep or rest in a completely horizontal position. I couldn't even sit on the sofa to rest. The rest required my head to be even with my heart to allow the blood to flow more easily.

Adrenal Management

The management of the adrenal is often tied into the management of thyroid issues. There are different approaches to the management of adrenal fatigue, one of which is to prevent some of the surges in the cortisol production related to stress. Another is to provide substrates for the production of hydrocortisone such as Pregnenolone.

A third approach is to suppress the breakdown of hydrocortisone and thus, higher levels from what is already being made. An example of that would be to use licorice root. If still low, one can take small physiological doses of hydrocortisone that are some fraction of what the adrenal gland normally would produce. Its normal production in a typical person might be about 20-40 mg per day. We usually give some fraction of that amount, in the morning, less at noon, and even less in the afternoon. This is an important point that most patients and physicians don't understand:

**As long as you give an amount that is
a small fraction of the total daily output of hydrocortisone,
then you are not likely to run into a complication
with regard to suppression of the adrenal gland
by the administration of extra hydrocortisone.**

Adrenal management for me was key in starting to feel like a real person again. It was reassuring to be able to take those small amounts to get through stressful or very busy days. It's not like taking amphetamines. I never felt "up" or a "high" I felt a little closer to normal. And on days that I was herxing or really low, nothing worked. My body knew it needed to rest and there was no argument to convince my body otherwise.

DR. MOZAYENI

Thyroid Hormone Management

One of the most common conditions I am able to clinically recognize and manage is euthyroid side syndrome, non-thyroidal illness syndrome or, aka, Hypothyroidism Type II. Most patients I see have all of the symptoms of hypothyroidism but have normal lab test results.

It is a controversy not unlike Lyme Disease as to whether or not you use the active form of thyroid hormone, Liothyronine T3 in the management of someone who is clearly suffering from all of the symptoms of hypothyroidism. Clinically it is obvious, but the labs don't corroborate it so physicians walk away from the patient and refuse to treat them. Even endocrinologist specialists do this all the time.

A patient who has chronic inflammation and small-vessel disease often will have impairment of their cellular metabolism so they develop a form of Hypothyroidism, at the cellular level. This type of patient needs T3 more than T4. This patient will often get sicker if given T4. Poor lab test methods and outdated laboratory science are to blame.

Patients' cells respond to the reduction of blood flow by conserving energy. One way this happens in the cell when it is impaired in its ability to receive nutrients, and oxygen, that it will internally adjusts the balance between T3 and reverse T3. At the cellular level in illness, these cells try to protect themselves by reducing their metabolic rate to conserve energy.

Other tissues in the body start reducing their energetics and then the muscle cell won't relax as well – this means that the muscles will tend to be tight or even in spasm. They also develop neurological and cognitive symptoms when they develop this form of hypothyroidism.

This form of hypothyroidism occurs at the cell or tissue level, not at the thyroid gland. It has to do with metabolism at the tissue level. They can have all the features of being hypothyroid without the lab results to prove it. This is exceedingly common in patients with chronic infections and small-vessel disease and thyroid lab tests are usually highly misleading.

Thyroid hormone management controversy is not quite as acrimonious as the Lyme controversy. The controversy is around whether or not to use T3, which is the active form of thyroid hormone.

While you are trying to get them better they do need extra support with T3. Usually, they do very poorly with Levothyroxine (T4) because it provides substrate for the further production of reverse T3 at the cellular level – but they do very well on T3. Of course there are concerns and precautions about how it is used and how often it is used. We all want to get the patient off of it as soon as we can but we also appreciate how helpful it is for the care and management of the patient.

It does require more effort on the part of the patient and practitioner in health cost-restrained times.

Ineffective/Outdated Testing

BH, T4, free T4, T3, free T3, and rT3 lab tests are all poor lab markers that should not be given priority over clinical findings in medical decision-making.

Outside the brain TSH moves to act on the thyroid gland, but it probably also acts on other tissues in the body. The TSH molecule has a protein backbone with a variety of different carbohydrate side groups. Depending on the patient's medical condition, the carbohydrate side chains on the TSH backbone can be modified to vary its effect on the thyroid gland itself and on the various tissues of the body.

I heard about this in 1986, a lecture given by Bruce Weintraub, MD, one of the NIH's experts in TSH, when I was a pre-doctoral HHMD Fellow at the NIH (National Institutes of Health). I immediately realized the measurements of TSH taken in a routine clinical laboratory are not reliable because they measure only the protein backbone. This lab test has not advanced in more than 20 years!

The lab measurements do not account for the variability of all the different side chains on the TSH molecule that then determine exactly what TSH really does. In a patient with chronic illness, that TSH molecule's function changes. It may even be causing a peripheral suppression of metabolism. There are many things TSH can do that we *should* be learning about but medical science is not presently pursuing this knowledge to improve thyroid function lab tests.

In patients with these chronic inflammatory states with vascular compromise and inflammation, the metabolic rate slows. Their cells do not get proper circulation. The cells do not receive adequate levels of oxygen, nutrients, and hormones. They do not remove the waste adequately, so the cells go into a state of lowered metabolism.

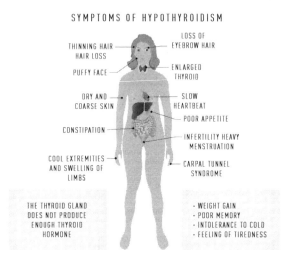

SYMPTOMS OF HYPOTHYROIDISM

THINNING HAIR
HAIR LOSS

LOSS OF
EYEBROW HAIR

PUFFY FACE

ENLARGED
THYROID

DRY AND
COARSE SKIN

SLOW
HEARTBEAT

POOR APPETITE

CONSTIPATION

INFERTILITY HEAVY
MENSTRUATION

COOL EXTREMITIES
AND SWELLING OF
LIMBS

CARPAL TUNNEL
SYNDROME

THE THYROID GLAND
DOES NOT PRODUCE
ENOUGH THYROID
HORMONE

· WEIGHT GAIN
· POOR MEMORY
· INTOLERANCE TO COLD
· FEELING OF TIREDNESS

As a result, the patient starts exhibiting all the manifestations of hypothyroidism clinically but with normal thyroid lab test results.

The thyroid tests and blood tests, with the exception of reverse

T3, are intended to measure the function of the thyroid gland. The body's responsiveness to the hormone produced by the thyroid gland, however, can vary depending on the level of circulation, inflammation, toxicity, etc. at the peripheral tissue level.

The current medical model is based on a simplistic assumption that the blood tests are all you need to measure because thyroid glandular function is the only thing you need to measure.

There simply is not any good, reliable technology to measure the way the body's tissue cells respond to thyroid hormone.

This is partly because we are not able to look at the details of how the carbohydrate side chains on the TSH molecules may be modified or rearranged depending on the patient's illness and partly because blood testing does not reflect intra-cellular T3 and rT3 balance.

SHARON

I went to the endocrinologist about two years prior for possible thyroid issues. My mother had suffered from thyroid issues from her early 30s onward. When I mentioned to her that I was losing a lot of my hair, my mother immediately suggested I go to an endocrinologist. My symptoms included:

- Depression
- Dry skin
- Hair loss, thinning and loss of eyebrows

- Increased sensitivity to cold and feeling cold all the time

- Fatigue

- Joint and muscle pain

- Mood swings

- Puffy face

- Rashes on skin

- Multiple food sensitivities

- Sensitivity to cold

- Weak fingernails

- Weight gain for no obvious reason

- Thickening of the skin

- Heavy menstrual flow or irregular periods

As most endocrinologists do, Dr. T went by the lab results. He diagnosed me with Hashimoto's Disease, but he was extremely conservative on prescribing medication.

Now, Dr. Mozayeni treats my adrenals and my thyroid in addition to the co-infections. I believe treating these two issues is critical to healing.

Euthyroid Sick Syndrome / Type II Hypothyroidism

In Endocrinology, as in any field of study, there are some concepts are poorly described, poorly understood and poorly taught. There is a concept called the euthyroid sick syndrome where the patient is sick but the test results are normal. This is described as something that is a transient state associated with, for example, viral illnesses or other issues. But to my knowledge there is no mention in any medical textbook of this being a persistent condition in patients with chronic inflammation, chronic infection, and chronic illness. However, the science of this was explained thoroughly in the Journal of Clinical Endocrinology and Metabolism (Koulouri Olympia, Moran Carla, et al. **Pitfalls in the measurement and interpretation of thyroid function tests**. *Best practice & research. Clinical endocrinology & metabolism.* December 2013; 27(6): 745–762 https://www.ncbi.nlm.nih.gov/pmc/articles/PMC3857600/).

My clinical experience has absolutely proven to me beyond any doubt whatsoever that this sort of euthyroid sick syndrome, which some refer to as Type II Hypothyroidism or thyroid resistance, is a very real and very important aspect of the care and management of a patient with chronic illness.

There is research related to the toxicities of thyroid hormone, overdosing or the toxicosis of an inflammatory thyroid condition such as Hashimoto's that has caused endocrinologists and others to be wary of using *any* dose of thyroid hormone for treatment. We are all taught the risks, dangers and symptoms of hyperthyroidism. In the setting of normal thyroid labs doctors are trained not to use any thyroid hormone, particularly T3. For these with chronic illness, this is unfortunate because T3 can jumpstart the dysfunctional metabolic pathways and alleviate many symptoms including brain fog. With better brain function and energy, the work of recovery becomes possible.

Myxedema

It is important in the evaluation of a chronically ill patient to look for and examine for a major sign of hypothyroidism, known as myxedema. Hypothyroidism has some other features as well, such as the

- thinning and coarsening of the hair,
- dryness and scaliness of the skin, and
- thinning of the outside edges of the eyebrows.

In patients with Hypothyroidism, the muscle relaxation rate is slowed, because the metabolic rate of the muscle is slowed. When you test the muscle reflexes at the biceps, forearm or Achilles tendon (calf inside) contraction, you can observe a delay in the relaxation rate after the rapid contraction phase. This can be measured in the forearm by a device called the Thyroflex. The Thyroflex is a mechanical device that actually measures the relaxation rate of the muscle and reports a number.

The concept here is to meet the needs of the patient rather than to worry about making the labs look right or to be guided by misleading lab results.

DR. MOZAYENI

The lab reports, at best, are a gauge of what the thyroid gland itself is doing. Despite concerns among endocrinologists regarding the risks of long-term excessive thyroid administration, when you manage a patient in this way you will not likely give them an excess dose. If you are monitoring their condition very carefully using all different modalities, it has been shown, even with long-term treatment, you don't ever permanently suppress TSH production by the pituitary. Even patients who have been on excessive T4 for decades can recover their TSH production within 1-2 weeks upon the withdrawal of thyroid hormone.

Connecting Adrenal and Thyroid Treatments

In patients with type II hypothyroidism, all of their tissues are metabolically suppressed, including their adrenals. Some adrenal function is required in order for the thyroid hormone to be able to up-regulate the metabolic rate. In patients who are adrenally fatigued, the administration of any thyroid hormone, even T3, will usually make them more tired, not less.

It is a well-known principle in functional medicine that you have to support the adrenals **before** you try to manage the hypothyroidism. You have to give patients a little adrenal support and get their energy level to improve before you can expect the thyroid hormone to have positive results. That is why in a typical patient, while we are waiting for all of the tests regarding their persistent infections, it helps to take a month or two to properly address the adrenal and thyroid aspects of their health. That way they can then better tolerate any potential anti-microbial therapy.

This functional aspect to the care of a patient with chronic illness is not one that many physicians who treat Lyme Disease will consider. Patients can become extremely sick and disabled if you try to treat them with some antibiotics; particularly those that will deplete their cortisol levels further; unless you first manage thyroid and adrenal function and get things in order. You need to help the patient become more functional and build more resiliency before starting antibiotic treatments.

PICC LINES

History of PICC Line Use

In this chapter, we will discuss the role of PICC (Peripherally Inserted Central Catheter) lines in the treatment of patients with Lyme Disease, including the risks and benefits as well as the justifications for using it or not using it.

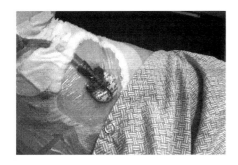

A central line is a way to get intravenous access that bypasses the peripheral veins so anything irritating or toxic to the veins can go into a larger blood vessel more centrally. Another reason to use a central line is to be able to give antibiotic therapies or other i.v. therapies over a long period of time. And, sometimes, the gut cannot be used so an i.v. line is needed.

Depending on where a central line is inserted, it may have to be changed every often to prevent infection. Whether you insert from the internal jugular or the arm to the brachial vein or via the subclavian vein under the clavicle, the purpose, from a therapy point of view is the same. You use the line to deliver concentrated, high doses of antibiotics or intravenous feedings centrally into a large vein. The idea of using a **peripherally** inserted central catheter became more of the norm because it was observed it could be left in for a much longer period of time. It was a relatively safe approach in that it went into the arm vein rather than in another vein, where during the process you could puncture the lung.

When treating Lyme Disease the PICC line is often used to provide long-term intravenous antibiotic therapy. The PICC line is a way to give patients high doses of intravenous antibiotics at home without having to change the line frequently.

Generally, these catheters have to be put in by a hospital-based invasive radiologist because they have to access a larger vein in the inside of the arm above the elbow above where blood is usually drawn. This keeps the line out of the way and allows them to tunnel the catheter under the skin for a few centimeters before it gets into the vein. This tunneling greatly reduces the risk of infection and line sepsis because it is protected under the skin, providing a greater barrier for infection to go from the surface of the skin down to the vein where it could spread.

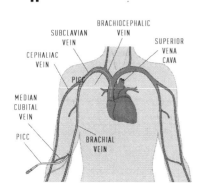

These catheters usually get infected from the skin surface. Skin hygiene, therefore, is important. The catheters have to be cleaned regularly. The skin surface near the catheter has to be cleaned regularly and a clear dressing is applied over it to protect the entry point and minimize the accumulation of bacteria. This is done to protect the catheter, the vein and the whole circulation and body from infection. This is why the PICC line can be left in for a much longer period of time than a central line put in through some other point.

Role of PICC Lines in Lyme Disease Treatment

Most doctors would agree with approved guidelines when it comes to using i.v. antibiotic therapy in Lyme Disease for a period of time when there is central nervous system involvement, or joint involvement unresponsive to oral antibiotics. We think of intravenous antibiotic therapy for Lyme Disease as being valid when:

- there is central nervous system involvement and/or
- there is significant joint involvement unresponsive to oral antibiotics.

The controversies around the PICC lines historically have developed around the duration of treatment. We are not going to get into that in this chapter. The duration of antibiotic therapy is a separate matter. The PICC line is a technological advance allows for relatively long durations of i.v. therapy.

The question really is, "Is it reasonable and appropriate to use a PICC line for long term antibiotics?" Many of these decisions are highly individualized. I don't think protocols should be used to force a template process on individuals – they need to be personalized.

Protocols are guidelines. Protocols have always been guidelines. And protocols should remain guidelines to allow individualized precision medicine.

This is a core concept of personalized medicine. The real challenge and controversy comes into deciding:

- how long to use the antibiotics i.v., and
- which antibiotics to use i.v.,

while considering facts such as germ resistance co-infections that may not have responded to the initial choice of antibiotics.

For the intravenous therapy of Lyme Disease, the classic i.v. antibiotic has been ceftriaxone. Other cephalosporins have been used as backup. There are other antibiotics available intravenously to treat *Borrelia* and other infections such as *Bartonella*. Some antibiotics are not available to be given intravenously. Some antibiotics penetrate cells so well they do not need to be given intravenously. They will penetrate quite well into cells and tissue when taken orally.

Another scenario in which PICC lines can be very helpful is if the patient has such a severe gastrointestinal problem; they simply cannot tolerate any oral antibiotic products. A PICC line may be a way to get the therapy started but once they get better, then they should switch over to oral antibiotic therapy. Personally, I have found it very rare to have a patient with a gut problem so severe you can't use oral antibiotic therapy. It is a rare scenario but it does happen.

Known Risks of a PICC Line

The known risks described on the Informed Consent forms range from phlebitis to infection, both, locally under the skin, or systemically along the catheter, into the vein and throughout the entire body. This can lead to endocarditis, an infection of the lining of the blood vessels including the heart valves, and it can lead to a stroke or even the need for valve replacement therapy.

The other risk of having a catheter is your body will probably will start coating it with biofilm. Fibrin deposits begin the formation of biofilm on the outside of the catheter on the part floating in the vein and the part tunneled under the skin.

When you put a catheter in, you always will get some fibrin coating, which may or may not grow large. A surface for biofilm to adhere to is then created. Then, some microbes may stick tightly to the biofilm on the catheter surface.

These biofilms may perpetuate the infection because the bacteria can then spread from the skin, track under the skin, along the catheter, into the vein, and along the catheter throughout its course into the central vein. If the fibrin layer grows, you can end up with a blood clot dangling on the end of a catheter. The blood clot can then break loose and float down the veins, go through the right chamber of the heart and end up in the lungs where it will cause a pulmonary embolism.

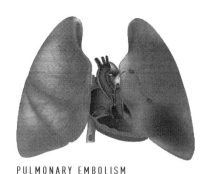

PULMONARY EMBOLISM

The pulmonary arterial circuit, which takes the venous blood from the body, acts as a filter also to trap small particles and small blood clots. Usually, those clots don't get to the other side of the circulation. There is a pathway normally open before birth, foramen ovale, but shortly after birth this opening closes. If it stays open it is called a patent foramen ovale (PFO).

In the adult population, a significant percentage of patients have a patent foramen ovale (PFO). A small clot or embolism on the venous side of the circulation can actually bypass the lungs and go into the left side of the circulation, go through the PFO and enter the left heart into the aorta through the arteries and land anywhere in the body including your brain where it would cause a stroke. It could also land in your kidney where it would cause an infarction. It could land in your muscles where it would cause a muscle infarction or transient muscle pain and tiny little showers of this stuff could end up causing significant neurovascular disease, cognitive impairment and even a dementia-like condition due to the all the micro-emboli flowing downstream to the brain.

There are some studies relating PFO to a higher risk of getting headaches and migraine headaches in particular. In a Lyme patient who has chronic headaches and various neurovascular symptoms to begin with, it is always a question as to whether or not they potentially have a PFO which would greatly increase their risk of an embolism, if they should be given a PICC line. It takes more testing to confirm a PFO – and this is not done routinely.

Other Risks of a PICC Line

That is one set of risks. The biofilm on the catheter is really interesting because germs form biofilms. When you have more than one germ in the circulation, as you usually do, you end up with colonies of different microbes in biofilms lining the blood vessels. The catheter also grows biofilms on itself and complicate anti-microbial therapy.

Biofilms are increasingly recognized as very important to scientists who study pharmacokinetics and who are concerned about the effectiveness of antibiotics and chemotherapy. They are concerned biofilms could potentially limit the effectiveness of the treatment. These biofilms, including the ones that can form on the catheter, could end up harboring the very bacteria that one is trying to treat with the antibiotics because you are inserting a foreign body, the catheter, into the system and letting your body coat it with fibrin and produce biofilm.

Any bacteria in the bloodstream could also be landing in the biofilm on the catheter and further contribute to the growth of the biofilms. The clots, thrombus and/or biofilm could end up breaking off while the catheter is in use or break off when the catheter is removed.

When a PICC line is removed there is always the potential for an acute pulmonary embolism. When we remove PICC line catheters, we want to do it very carefully and with supervision including a measurement of the oxygen saturation just in case.

Indirect Risks of a PICC Line

There is another very important indirect risk when using a PICC line. The peripherally inserted central catheter is a foreign body. The medical community treats fevers in a patient who has with a foreign body differently than a patient who does not have a foreign body. When you have a PICC line it changes the way the health care system approaches you when you have a fever; the intensity of the response is likely to be much higher.

Regardless of why you have a fever, whether from having the flu, or some other infection, the medical system has a set of rules and guidelines, safety measures, to first make sure you don't have catheter line-related sepsis; that you don't have systemic spread of infection from the catheter that could hurt you badly, or even kill you.

If you have a fever and have to go to the hospital, the typical protocol, regardless of the fever, is to immediately remove the catheter, culture the tip, draw blood cultures and make sure the individual does not have a catheter-related infection. A new catheter is then put in either at the same time or later, once that infection is ruled out. If another central line is put in, that central line carries its owns risks. If it is put in centrally, through the subclavian, there is a risk of puncturing the lung and that creates major complications, which may require a chest tube and a substantial stay in the hospital.

Once you are in the hospital you can have hospital-type accidents happen to you. You can get other infections from being in a hospital, like MRSA, Methicillin Resistant *Staphylococcus Aureus*, or you can get the wrong medication administered to you by accident. The potential for error is always there; the more you have done to you in a setting where intense treatments are administered, i.e. in a hospital, you can potentially end up being given the wrong drug or have some sort of nosocomial infection or what we call an iatrogenic illness. These are infections you get from being in a health care institution or medical injuries that you might get from being in an environment where something bad can happen to you accidentally. Your practitioners and your caregivers have to be vigilant. Most importantly, if you develop a complication, those caregivers need to be very careful it doesn't lead to more severe complications.

The risk versus benefit calculus is a very important consideration in the decision as to whether or not to put in the PICC line.

Some of the risks are obvious, some are subtle, but very important. I think many are often dismissed as being insignificant when I don't think they are insignificant at all. I think they are very real.

From what I have seen I think the risk of a PICC line is much higher than people realize. I also believe biofilm can get on the catheter and potentially harbor the very bacteria you are trying to treat. You could be giving the antibiotic therapy, all the while, there is more bacteria growing on the PICC line resistant to your antibiotic.

To understand what happens to germs in biofilm, consider that a biofilm is a bit like a thick gel. If you have an antibiotic on one side of the gel it may not diffuse adequately into the biofilm. The germs may be in a hard-to-penetrate space in the biofilm protected from the antibiotic. When germs are protected this way, they may appear to be resistant. They may not be resistant at all; they may be in a protected environment not getting exposed to effective concentrations of antibiotic even when it's being given intravenously.

Typically the doses of antibiotics used intravenously are not much higher than those prescribed orally. Sometimes, they are even lower so the total dose is often about the same. With i.v. antibiotics, you do get a sharper and higher increase in blood concentration for a shorter period of time. If you give it orally it might be absorbed more slowly. You may not get the same high blood levels but you can get reasonably good levels. If the gut is handling it you can increase the oral dose to get even better blood levels of antibiotics. If the antibiotics are ones that have to penetrate tissue in order to work, then they also tend to be well absorbed from the gut.

Let's go through some scenarios for specific germs to make these points even more clear. If you are treating *Borrelia*, the usual antibiotic is a cephalosporin called Ceftriaxone. Different standards of care exist as to whether or not you would need additional antibiotic therapy besides this cephalosporin. Some people believe you should give a form of tetracycline like Doxycycline or Minocycline. Some physicians believe other forms of bacteria, such as cyst forms must be addressed, so Flagyl might be prescribed as well. These are all areas of controversy and a lot of the thinking around the use of more antibiotics for *Borrelia* has been due to the fact that many patients don't respond to the first tier of antibiotics prescribed for treatment.

There are other explanations for patients not responding to the first tier of antibiotics. The patient may have a totally different microbe than what is initially diagnosed. It is possible that bands on the Western blot test showing up as slightly positive for *Borrelia* are actually cross reacting to other bacteria, such as *Bartonella.* That sort of cross-reaction can cause some false positive results for *Borrelia* on the Western blot test.

Finally, with Lyme Disease you may have blood-borne *Protozoa* such as *Babesia*. It is thought of as a co-infection, but recent emerging clinical research and experience indicates there may be varieties of *Protozoa*, from various different families other than *Babesia*. They can vary considerably. We are only now beginning to realize the situation is more complicated than we thought.

If this is true, and it certainly seems to be, then a single-minded approach to using high-dose antibiotic therapy for *Borrelia* via a PICC line may be totally off-base if these other infections are the dominant players and the dominant contributors to the symptoms.

If *Protozoa* or *Bartonella* are significant and are contributing in large part to the patient's symptoms, then a high-intensity *Borrelia* approach using a PICC line, (just because someone is not responding to the first-tier antibiotics), is going to be the wrong approach and will likely fail while increasing risk.

Antibiotics for Co-infections

Let's look at the co-infections and what antibiotics might treat them. In the case of *Bartonella*, we need to think about the principles of antibiotic therapy. Antibiotics are either *bactericidal*, which means that they immediately kill the germ or *bacteriostatic,* which means that they prevent it from growing. Bacteriostatic antibiotics prevent a germ from reproducing, but do not kill the germ. Eventually, the germ will reach the end of its life cycle and die on its own and/or the immune system is given an opportunity to take it over. It cannot resist the immune system when it is compromised by a bacteriostatic antibiotic.

Bartonella can move into a cell to escape antibiotics. They can move into a red cell when exposed to antibiotics outside the red cell. They will prefer to be on the outside of the red cell and in the circulation or attached to endothelial cells. But when you give antibiotics of any kind, if you give antibiotics for *Borrelia,* you can and will drive the *Bartonella* into the cells where it will escape your antibiotic. Therefore, you have to use antibiotics that can penetrate into the cell.

One antibiotic that may be bactericidal for *Bartonella* can be given only by the intravenous (i.v.) route. However, this antibiotic may penetrate cells very well. So if you have *Bartonella* and you think you are treating it, there is really no good role for i.v. antibiotic therapy. If an antibiotic is too toxic to make it of long-term use and if it does not get into cells, then it is not going to ultimately work very well. That adds to the risk of the PICC line. Thus, for this antibiotic, there is only a narrow window in an extremely sick person who cannot tolerate antibiotics by mouth.

Because there is ambiguity about which germs are actually causing the symptoms and because we know *Bartonella* can escape by moving into cells when necessary, it can escape some antibiotic therapies. And because the antibiotic therapies for *Bartonella* are bacteriostatic, not bactericidal, we have to rely more on the duration of therapy being adequate rather than being obsessed with achieving high intravenous doses.

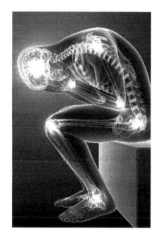

Patients who have *Bartonella* and receive antibiotic therapy usually develop a lot of joint and muscle pain within 10-14 days. Theoretically, if you go at it really hard and fast intravenously, you can potentially make the patient very uncomfortable, if not very ill, by approaching them with a high intensity of intravenous therapy. We now know *Bartonella* is a big player in patients with the symptoms of Lyme Disease and only the exceptional patient may need intravenous therapy. This changes the thinking about how to treat patients with Lyme Disease. If the majority of their symptoms are actually from circulatory disturbances caused by the endothelial infections associated with *Bartonella*, various *Protozoa* and the biofilms of these germs impairing the microcirculation, then the focus of therapy needs to be as much or more on those things than it should be on the *Borrelia* itself and i.v. antibiotic use should be reserved for more extreme circumstances.

Risk vs. Benefit Equation

We have to acknowledge the importance of the microcirculation (the biofilm, *Bartonella*, *Protozoa*).

Our clinical experience suggests that more often the symptoms seem to be caused by these other germs and less so by the *Borrelia* itself.

This changes the equation about the risks versus the potential benefits of using PICC lines for the treatment of *Borrelia* itself.

The public, lay definition of Lyme Disease is a very broad term that may or may not specifically be related to the presence of *Borrelia*. With any of these chronic infections, we don't have a way of knowing what is actually causing the symptoms except through significant clinical experience. Truthfully, even then, we really can't be too certain.

As stated earlier, the term #Lyme Disease is a very broad catch-all for a wide range of potential chronic infections ranging from *Borrelia* to *Bartonella* to *Babesia* to various other *Protozoa* and the biofilms they produce and the microcirculation they impair.

One has to look at the overall therapeutic approach and ask the question, "What priority should you give the intensity of *Borrelia* treatment with a PICC line relative to the attention you need to pay to the presence of these other co-infections, the *Protozoa*, the *Bartonella*, the biofilms and the circulatory problems they cause?" The physician needs to decide how much emphasis to give the treatment using the PICC line versus everything else. The recent emergence of technology allows us for the first time to see in #Lyme Disease (as defined by the public) the true prevalence of *Bartonella* and the true prevalence of the various *Protozoa*.

A high-dose intravenous antibiotic approach for *Borrelia* is misplaced when that patient has a multitude of symptoms that could very well stem primarily from a variety of co-infections. In my experience, this is the case in most #Lyme Disease patients.

As the science has evolved, and the understanding of *Bartonella*, *Protozoa*, biofilms, and microcirculation have all evolved, the role for intravenous antibiotic therapy for *Borrelia* seems to be diminishing. This is why I have shifted my approach. I have found my present 'co-infection'-focused approaches without PICC lines to be far more effective than when I was using PICC lines for intravenous treatment of Borreliosis specifically.

TREATING
FAMILY MEMBERS
SIMULTANEOUSLY

Dr. Mozayeni prefers to take family members under treatment separately. Through the difficult phases, a single patient's treatment can be very stressful within the family; treating more than one can exacerbate the stress. Treatment is time consuming, energy draining, and at times daunting. Setting up medication schedules and pillboxes can take an hour a week for each patient. Medications can alter a patient's taste buds, so meals might have to change. And the herxes can throw everyone's schedules off from getting laundry done to needing quiet time in the house.

From One Family Member to Two

When I started in September of 2009, we had no plans to test Jeff or Stephen until "later."

Two months later, Stephen developed those multiple infections (sinus, ear, strep, bronchitis) and his Lyme test was CDC-positive. His *Bartonella* titers were among the highest Dr. Mozayeni had seen thus far in his practice. Stephen had three strains of *Bartonella*. We initiated treatment immediately.

Looking back, I suspect Stephen was born with *Bartonella*, and that it was transmitted in utero. Unknown to us until very shortly after his birth, Stephen had a congenital birth defect, and it required immediate surgery the same day as he was born. The surgery was successful, but a few days later, one lung collapsed, necessitating a chest tube insertion.

For years after, Stephen battled recurrent bouts of pneumonia accompanied by low-grade intermittent fevers. He was hospitalized several times for the pneumonia. He later also contracted mononucleosis twice. We assumed it was all related to his birth defect and resulting surgery. We had no idea *Bartonella* was in play. I can't prove *Bartonella* was the cause, but I know once Stephen completed treatment, his bouts of pneumonia and low-grade fevers ended.

Starting Stephen into treatment during mine, I didn't know what we were in for. Fortunately, Dr. Mozayeni did. He kept me on my antibiotics, but instead of adding the more difficult treatment, he put me on a gentler treatment to help stay the bacteria while we started Stephen on treatment. Dr. Mozayeni was keenly sensitive to keeping the family unit cohesive and on an even keel. The stress levels easily rise during treatment due sometimes to increased pain, increased presentation of symptoms, including fear and anxiety.

Stephen's energy levels plummeted as we tried to get him through the third and fourth quarters of his junior year. A student usually works the hardest in the junior year, trying to look especially appealing to the colleges. Stephen spent his year trying to gain the energy to stay upright throughout the school day. He came home and slept, with no energy or stamina to work on homework or study for tests.

I wrote emails to his teachers explaining *Bartonella*, the treatment process, and the side effects of medications. Luckily, most of Stephen's teachers were compassionate and willing to work with us. At a time when most parents were urging their children to push harder, Jeff and I were simply proud of the fact that Stephen could make it through each school day without collapsing before 2:30 pm.

Stephen got through the worst of his treatment by the end of the school year. My turn was next. I started the more intense phase of treatment on July 5, 2010. July and August are the slowest months for my business. It was the best time for me to miss workdays if required. I was grateful for the timing aspect as I was able to work only about three to four hours a day before having to come home and get horizontal in bed to rest.

All in the Family

With Stephen and me undergoing treatment, we decided to take the leap and have Jeff tested. He tested positive for one strain of *Bartonella*.

Jeff started into treatment that fall, as I was coming out of the worst of it. Staggering the medication start dates for each family member was essential for us. We needed one individual who could manage laundry, meals, and errands. If we had all gone on it at the same time, it would have been disastrous and even more stressful for everyone.

It is not easy to be in treatment together. For us, however, it did work to our benefit.

With all three of us having *Bartonella*, we developed a sense of camaraderie that might not otherwise exist. When I started into the toughest phase of treatment and experienced my first bout of deep bone pain, Stephen sat next to me, put his arm around me, and said, "Hang in there, Mom. I promise you, this will pass and you will start to feel better. It doesn't feel like this all the time."

Wait – isn't it supposed to be the parent who says this to the child? Probably. But the tables were turned and I was grateful for his reassurance and positive attitude. I needed it desperately. Stephen was my role model for healing. Whether or not that's the way it's "supposed to be" that's what it was and I am grateful he was there for me.

When Jeff's herxes (side effects from the meds) manifested later, Stephen and I were able to validate his experience and remind him it was temporary and would eventually pass. While intellectually, every patient probably knows the pain won't last, it is comforting to hear those words repeated in the midst of the pain and frustration.

SHARON

Healing Times Vary

The only warning I would give is to watch for an increasing frustration level when one family member is not healing as "quickly" as the others. I started treatment two months before Stephen and six months before Jeff. But both of them completed their respective treatment in 16-18 months. I was very happy they were done, but I was very frustrated with my own seemingly slow progress.

Dr. Mozayeni compassionately reminded me I had been sick for 30 years. They had been sick for less time. And, **children heal faster and better than adults**. The infection had insidiously permeated almost every part of my body; it would simply take longer and more meds to obliterate it. Intellectually, I understood this. Emotionally, I cried on some of my trips home from the doctor. I wanted to be better *now*.

How Did We Get Through It?

Other Lyme patients have asked Jeff and me how we got through it. I often respond, "not very gracefully!" Some times were obviously better than others. We are not the poster children for this disease, that's for sure.

Here are some elements of what we agree did work for us:

ACCEPTANCE —To have the entire family diagnosed and treated at the same time is extremely stressful. But for us, it worked. We each understood the pain and energy it took to heal. We knew what each other was going through. Even though each family member had a different set of symptoms, we could empathize with each other.

AGREE TO DISAGREE AND THEN **LET GO** WITH **LOVE** –The old saying is, "Do you want to be right or do you want to be happy?" Sometimes we didn't agree on how or when to do things. So, we disagreed and respected one another's opinions and moved forward. Resentment does not aid in healing.

BEST FRIENDS – Jeff and I were best friends when we married. We had almost 20 years of marriage when this diagnosis hit our family. Being best friends was essential in maintaining respect, admiration, and enjoying hanging out with one another.

CHOOSE YOUR BATTLES – This one was critical with raising Stephen. He was a junior in high school; when most students are working on their hardest classes, preparing for colleges, our son was trying not to fall asleep in class while getting through the roughest part of the protocol. Life got down to the basics. But it was not a classic teenage angst filled year. It was a year of trying to heal: simple as that.

COMPASSION – with all of us being sick, we were less likely to be angry when the laundry wasn't done, or the dishwasher wasn't unloaded, or when we ordered pizza for the third time that week. There was very little judgment on each of our parts because we all knew how terrible the meds and/or the disease could make us feel.

DATING – Jeff and I still go out on dates with one another. Sometimes, it's coffee or ice cream in the afternoon. It's whatever we can manage. But it's a time and space for us to enjoy each other's time and company. It's a time to remember why we started liking each other in the first place. With Stephen it's lunch or coffee or shopping for school. It's one-on-one time, where we can chat and catch up with no set agenda.

DON'T TAKE IT PERSONALLY – Jeff used to think I forgot his grocery items on purpose. It took awhile, and a lot of my showing him times when I forgot things important to other people or to me. He finally realized I wasn't doing things "at" him. I was sick. And because he was the closest person to me, he often bore the brunt of my symptoms.

ENCOURAGEMENT – When things are looking up, acknowledge it, celebrate it. Every bit of encouragement helps everyone.

FUN – No matter how small, find ways to have fun with each other. Sometimes, we went to a farmer's market for 45 minutes and that was it for the weekend. But we enjoyed it together and it helped us bond even more.

LAUGHTER – It's important to laugh with each other, not at each other; important to watch funny television shows together; to pick up the slack when the other is feeling down.

MARRIAGE COUNSELING WHEN NECESSARY – Sometimes you need a third party to help. It's not easy and it's not fun, but it is part of what saved our marriage during a real rough patch.

PROBLEM SOLVING – Going up and down stairs became impossible for me. For Christmas, Jeff installed a smaller washer and dryer unit off our bathroom so I no longer needed to make trip up and down. It has been one of the most thoughtful, kindest gifts he has ever given me.

SPIRITUAL FOUNDATION – We both have a similar spiritual foundation. We both have the same "starting point." We both believe in the power of prayer and we prayed a lot.

TEAMWORK – When I was diagnosed, Jeff started an organic garden for me. He encouraged me to start eating only organic foods. He educated me on how to change my diet. But then he let me make those changes at my own pace. He didn't force it down. He let me find my path alongside his. When he started keeping bees to help pollinate the garden and to give us raw, unfiltered honey, I didn't do much with the bees, but I help him fill the bottles and put the labels on them.

EFFECTS OF INTERNET AND TECHNOLOGY

DR. MOZAYENI

Technology Trends

The more we study the biochemistry of the human body, the more information there is, so it becomes a huge challenge for any one individual to even think about mastering all there is to know. Over

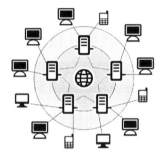

the past 20 years, physicians have increasingly specialized in their practices; their credibility has been a very deep narrow expertise rather than broad systems integration expertise. Depth is traded for the breadth.

Let's return to the old medical school newsletter cartoon I referred to earlier in this book. "As physicians progress through internship, residency and then specialty, they learn more and more about less and less, until we know a lot about very little." It takes experience to build breadth with depth.

We have now moved to an era where everything other than the most routine issue is always associated with an Internet search. That transition, that access to information, is no longer entirely in the hands of the clinician. A patient can also access much of the same information. But the patient must also have a need, the time to search, and the composure, physiology and brain function to allow them to search for and comprehend the information.

Elsewhere in this book, we covered issues involving Internet research and the problems it can raise. If you take a look on the Internet for opinions about what to do for Lyme Disease, you will find little agreement about what should be done. The agreements or the consensus only start to build if you take a one-sided view as seen by one side of the controversy.

We have access to content produced by many people with a desperate – people need who don't typically have the medical and scientific training to be able to discern the wheat from the chaff.

For those reasons and because the treatments and the diagnostic pathways have not been working reliably in the world of Lyme Disease, the public has been using every imaginable form of standard and alternative treatments in the treatment of Lyme Disease. They have resorted to any number of diagnostic tests believing or not believing findings, depending on perspective.

People mostly cannot use a scientific filter to understand a test result is rarely, if ever, a certainty; it is always a probability. It's like looking at a blurry image. If the image was perfectly clear you might see something, but most test results are not so clear. And so much of the data is based on anecdotal experiences.

If you look at the public posts on the Internet, you can see clear biases in posts on the Internet. These biases fall into a few categories.

One category is the posting from the patient who had a treatment and is feeling great about it. One of two things is likely to happen.

First, they may post about it but then they will drop off because they are fine and they want to get back to their life. So there is this little nugget of information and then it's gone.

Second, the person has such a great result they actually overdo it, they start talking about it too much. They talk about it so much it dilutes out any other possible dialogue. Others, in their hope of finding a better answer, end up trying that treatment not realizing it only worked for them.

There is this incredible need, desperation really, for people to be able to compare themselves to one another medically. There are patterns emerging in how people respond with a disease as a result of the various potential chronic infections.

But there is enough variability in an individual's genetic makeup, the ways the genes are expressed (called the phenotype), also their diet, nutrition, living environment, psychosocial stressors, and a variety of other lifestyle factors – that make it very, very difficult, if not impossible, to compare one person to another.

Despite the clinician's best efforts to explain this, patients still want to go back and compare notes with others to see how they are doing.

Often, I will prescribe a set of highly individualized treatments and it completely escapes the patient how individualized it is. Later, you learn they've blogged it and are asking the world of non-medical people for their opinion about the set of treatments their physician just prescribed.

But then I realize there is a certain beauty to what is actually happening. There is this incredible need to share experiences, to get any kind of information at all from anyone else's experience and there is occasional some credibility in other people's opinions about their treatments.

What people are doing is called "checking behavior." We check with each other to see, "Is your experience like mine? Is this in the range of 'normal?'"

Patients need to have "buy-in," and especially in our western culture that means they have to take part in deciding their "preferred" course of treatment. We are that into self-determination, insofar as is possible.

Patient Preference

If you look at evidence-based medicine and the academic writings related to evidence-based medicine, patient preference is critical because patient preference determines the perception of benefit and harm. I believe most patients searching the Internet are really trying to find all they can to fully inform them – to have the full informed consent conversation from a perspective they can't possibly get from the clinician.

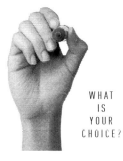

WHAT
IS
YOUR
CHOICE?

While we know this goes on, almost all patients still tend to follow the physician's program; they want this information but they still will do what they are asked to do most of the time. I have seen many situations in which the patient hesitates because of something they've heard and that is fine. I don't think anyone should be putting something in their body unless they feel comfortable doing so because even if it is right for all the right medical reasons it still can have a "nocebo effect" – the opposite of a placebo effect.

I constantly tell people, "It's very important for you to feel comfortable with what you are taking. It doesn't matter if your concern about it is rational or irrational; you still have to be comfortable doing it." I think it is incredibly important to help patients stay centered as they recover.

As a clinician, I realize this is not about my deciding what is best for my patient. The days of the paternalistic medical model are gone except for emergencies in which the patient doesn't meet the criteria of being physically and mentally able, or because of urgency, have enough time to analyze their predicament and influence it. In a true medical emergency that lands you in an emergency room you really don't have time to do so. But in almost every other situation I think this Internet-based "check-in" consent model is the right model and in the future it may become the only model, because of the Internet.

The Internet has been a major game changer because it is the first comprehensive way to get information and all perspectives.

Information Trends

Along with the Internet we have two major trends. One is better communication through email and all kinds of social media: Facebook, Twitter, blogs, where there are snippets of information going out – basically verbal data being exchanged between individuals asynchronously but more or less in real time.

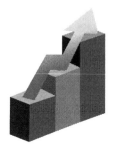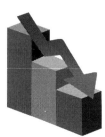

The second trend is the availability of information in the databases holding all the information, and the analysis of the data in those systems, is referred to as big data. The promise of big data is that with computers you can sort out the messiness of real world data to glean useful information.

When you are managing a case, you have to remember that guidelines are not rules or laws – only suggestions that may be outdated. When a treatment is not working, when it is failing, you have to refine your hypothesis and consider other possibilities, however unlikely they may be.

The following is a particular case I was recently involved with. One case of Juvenile Arthritis, the parents, because the child's treatment was failing and there was a history of Lyme Disease, sought out advice and support from people who had experience with Lyme Disease – including patients and physicians. The parents realized there were potential underlying co-infections to be considered.

When the child was originally diagnosed and treated for Lyme Disease no one ever looked at co-infections. The presumption was the patient's condition had deteriorated because either there was an impartial or incomplete treatment of Lyme Disease or there was a co-infection, or really an infection unrelated to Lyme Disease, that they might have gotten from exposure to *Bartonella* from a cat or from a flea or a *Protozoan* infection from a mosquito.

The parents sought out the care of more expert clinicians. In doing so, they wanted to synergize these other approaches for the child's treatment for the autoimmune condition with other approaches; particularly, approaches more restorative than immune suppressive. They were trying to rescue their child who had become crippled as a result of all these immune suppressive treatments and her underlying diagnosis of juvenile arthritis.

Because the parents wanted to deviate from the standard of care, the physician managing the case reported the parents to government Child Protective Services. As the parents were seeking out better information to try to take care of their child and struggling with their child's illness, the purveyor of the standard of care approach is reporting them for failure to follow his provided care plan and potentially putting the child's life in danger. That particular clinician's training and experience was mostly in managed care and/or in institutions in a state where the medical establishment and the government were both hostile to the diagnosis of Lyme Disease.

Through information access (it can be a phone call, Internet and ultimately better advice through big data coming back and informing patient decision-making and clinician decision-making), the shared model of responsibility becomes the only viable model and a basis for comprehensive informed consent. <u>A patient or clinician who fails to acknowledge this will get into trouble.</u> It's really the only ethical and rational way.

Practitioner and patient need to have open communication and consider broadly, without bias, all available options in a model of shared responsibility.

Unfortunately, all of this requires long office appointments. And, some part of the appointment is going to have to deal with the potential information toxicity one gets from plugging your brain into the Internet. There will be nuggets of good information here and there and better tools over time helping us to make better decisions, but the tools will always be less than perfect. There will always be some chaff, some Internet information toxicity, together with related confusion and anxiety along with the opportunity.

The broad trend here is the democratization of health care. It is empowering individuals with the information they need served up in a way they understand driven by a combination of experts looking at big data to make sure it can provide useful actionable information for individuals.

There are other trends that also speak to this. There are other movements. One of them is called personalized medicine. There is a group called the Personalized Medicine Coalition. The goal is to find treatment that works for you in any situation, not just for the condition in every patient. The National Institutes of Health (NIH) has a large precision medicine initiative with tremendous potential.

Again the goal is similar; to recognize and find better technologies for individualized care. In fact, there is a group of scientists, citizens and investors, who are very much focused on trying to develop technologies to help individualize care, such as specific genomic technologies. But recognize that these genomic technologies are enabled by information systems. That is called Computational Biology.

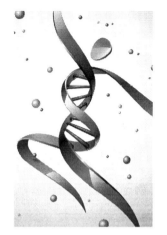

The ability we now have to sequence the human genome is the direct result of computational power. It starts with DNA you hit with specific enzymes. As though with a shotgun, the enzymes will blast the DNA into millions of different irregular pieces. Then, with the help of computers you sequence every fragment. Because there is an overlap among all the fragments, the computer can also solve the puzzle of what pieces go in what order. You have the sequence data (which is a mess) and then the computer actually solves the puzzle of how the puzzle pieces fit together.

It can solve the puzzle because you actually give it a thousand different versions of the same puzzle. You have the cut lines of the puzzle occurring in many different ways. You give the computer a thousand different ones and it can solve a thousand puzzles at once in order to answer the question of what is the picture in the puzzle. At this time you can probably get your entire genome sequenced for about $5,000.

When we run a *Bartonella* test, if it is positive, we are certain about the result because the isolated DNA is submitted through the same kind of sequencing to prove that the DNA fragment is in fact from *Bartonella*. The entire sequence of the *Bartonella* microbe is determined so we can confirm it is in fact a strain of *Bartonella* and not simply a piece of it.

Traditional Mainstream Medicine

If you are getting information through the Internet it is as much in real time as anything can be. When you do a Google search you don't necessarily know what data is current or relative. Some things are dated; some things are not. There is always a question of whether or not it is relevant to you; is it the most relevant or the newest thought about something. In traditional, mainstream medicine, we are following clinical standards 20 to 50 years old because it takes 17 to 20 years for adoption of any kind of new approach.

By definition everyone is kind of running around employing the protocols from the mainstream medical communities. These institutional healthcare systems and managed care models are all predicated on protocols often 20 or more years old. Most cannot keep up with the newest information, which is one of the reasons I don't think they work optimally.

With the Internet you can access real-time information, so you expect faster innovation – ultimately, the big 'win' here. Now we can all innovate faster. But innovation occurs in pockets and in leaps of various sizes. One clinician may be innovative in one area but it can take time to reach the point where it can be written down as a protocol and published.

The process has been slow and here is why:

1. In the standard medical innovation model you may receive a grant a year or two after applying for it.
2. You start your study (which can take a year to initiate).
3. The study runs two to three years.
4. It takes another six to twelve months to analyze the data and write the paper.
5. Then it can take another three to twelve months to get the paper through the editors and the reviewers and get it published.
6. Then it lands in paper form on a bookshelf in a library and a privately owned journal locks that information down with a copyright.

Millions of federally funded dollars of research money (public money) went into creating an article that sits in a copyright vault whether it is online or in a library. It is not presented to physicians. It is not incorporated into the standard of care – instead, it just sits there.

If I am pioneering a protocol for *Bartonella* or *Protozoa* or *Borrelia* or anything else, it takes time to get it to the point where it would be medically or ethically responsible to write it down and put it out for everyone to use. We need to be certain about it and describe it in reproducible detail. Even in the best of all worlds, it could take a good two years.

This point completely and utterly escapes people on the Internet because they are desperately seeking new information. They don't realize they are getting more access to the most recent ideas, untested protocols. Because most readers have never been in scientific research, they don't realize that you have to bake the idea, test it, replicate it yourself, ask your colleagues to replicate it and then even try to disprove it, before publishing it. If you are making a cake you've got to bake it before you start serving it.

Medical innovation on the Internet has many pitfalls.

A responsible innovator will be careful about publicizing suggestions or protocols and only then do so after they have personally tried to disprove their own theory or recommendation.

Same Meds, Different Dosages

You can give one drug in a different way to different people and it can cause dramatically different results. Most physicians have forgotten their most basic lessons in pharmacokinetics. You have to understand the concept of the drug half-life. You have to understand the difference between peak blood level and trough level. The trough levels and peak levels determine the toxicity and efficacy of the drug.

For example, if you use two antibiotics simultaneously, you must consider that they absorb at different rates. You have to be careful whether you dose it with food or without food. The timing affects drug levels and thus determines the effects and side effects.

It is almost futile for the layperson to try to sort this out. Ninety percent of physicians cannot sort it out. How do you expect the lay public who never took a course in pharmacology to be able to sort this out <u>and</u> to do it while they are anxious and cognitively impaired?

Healthcare Fail

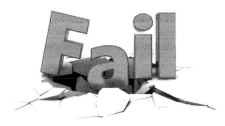

Sadly, the desperation is often driven by a people with chronic illness, navigating in a failed health care system. Many of them live hours away from any urban center. Even if they could find a practitioner where they are, it would be hard for them to convince that person to treat them. Patients often feel they are on their own and some even try to get medications from their veterinarians. If they raise cattle they try to get it from their cattle feed supplier. A lot of people are, either by geography or by their finances or by their other circumstances, unable to access to the right kind of care.

Most patients start off with their mainstream doctors who vary greatly in skill and compassion levels for that patient's specific condition. Those mainstream practitioners usually participate with insurance companies; meaning, they are restricted by the insurance company in terms of the services they may render.

The practitioners' client becomes the insurance company, not the patient.

Read that again: **the practitioners' client becomes the insurance company, not the patient.**

Practitioners cannot innovate and they cannot deviate.

The standardization and inter-connection of electronic health records create a greater risk of centralized control and limitation of care and innovation to depersonalize personalized medicine.

By law, all physicians and all health care entities now have a National Provider Identification number, the NPI number. The NPI number is like a doctor's professional Social Security Number. Every test they order, every drug they order, whether it's an x-ray or an antibiotic, is now tracked in a big data system under this NPI number. Every single health care interaction is now tracked.

Thus, many clinicians live in fear of what their institution or their group practice or what national health care panels might say about what they do. It is going to get to the point where, as they are entering an order in their electronic data system, in their computer, they will get flags and warnings telling them to do or not do something. And guess who is going to be writing those algorithms? The insurance companies.

Managed care is going to be writing those policies. The Federal organizations outsource these policies; almost all of Medicare administration is outsourced to private companies. Region by region, whoever gets the contract for that year can determine exactly how the policies are implemented unless there is a national coverage determination.

Constitutionally, healthcare Is in the governance of the States and not in the Federal domain. The Federal government became involved once they chose to tax and pay for the services. It needs to come back to the States because there is too much regional variability and need. Healthcare has to be local. It needs to be individualized and personalized and it needs to occur at the individual level.

Ultimately, I have confidence that big data will bring about the full and proper personalization, care and help medical innovation but it's going to take 10-20 years to get past the political and business controls on health care to the point of allowing the data to speak for itself.

Remember, the insurers are not actually the insurance companies. The employer is the insurer in the case of large companies; they decide the policy benefits and what goes in it and what gets covered. If they realize there is a better way to use big data to provide more efficient and effective care to individuals at a cheaper price with a better workforce, you can bet it will happen. The question is how do we get there and how many people will suffer until we get there?

It is not in the best interest of employers to spend money on the care of the chronically ill. Government healthcare has supported this position and even in the Affordable Health Care Act, has not made any commitment to adopting innovation in healthcare.

In an ideal world, the Internet data coming in real time would to be analyzed scientifically and moderated, quelling a lot of the anxiety and concern in Internet forums. Currently, much of what you see on various social media sites and blogs contains speculation and anxiety. I don't think it's going to change but I think that we can encourage our patients to go into secured private forums, where there are members following ground rules. Many large social media companies have created these free-for-all blogs so they can have viewer eyeballs on the page. The crazier the stuff that is said on the blog the more eyeballs go on the page.

Most people don't realize why Google is free. Yes, you get a free search but they learn about everything you look for. Basically, they give you some data for free while you give them some incredibly priceless access to you. Beware of the free data services.

People on the Internet Asking Technical Questions

Many people on the Internet blogs are not seeking technical or medical information. They may think they are but often, they are simply trying to allay their anxiety. They are actually trying to distract themselves from their anxiety and their emotional and spiritual needs by trying to ask technical questions about non-existent protocols. Patients with these chronic illnesses are suffering from a microbe and its ravages. They are often suffering from other things that make them vulnerable to the microbe's causing illness. The germ is one part of the puzzle but the terrain, the body and the way they respond to the germ, is the other.

You can take two people in a similar situation confronting, let's say, a bad guy on the street. One guy will find a nuance way to side-skirt a potential conflict and the other one may start a gunfight. The outcome has nothing to do with the guy they ran into, it has to do with how they responded to the guy they ran into. The same is true with these illnesses. The fact that a patient is obsessing over some microbe is often an underlying significant psychological disturbance and possibly a personality disorder.

According to an article published in the New England Journal of Medicine in the 1990s, between 11-36 percent of all general care physician visits involved patients with diagnosable psychiatric disorders (L. Eisenberg, "Treating depression and anxiety in primary care", New England Journal of Medicine, 1992, 326). When there are underlying personality disorders and psychiatric issues, instead of confronting it, patients will put the blame on something else like a microbe. This is why treating a chronically ill patient is significantly more complicated than anyone will give it credit for.

I am **NOT** saying Lyme Disease is a personality disorder. This is very important. The way you respond to an illness and the way you conduct yourself in seeking your care can be and often is the result of your personality and your psychological predispositions. And these disorders can result from infections causing mental illness!

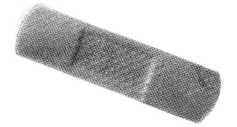

When people have an emotionally traumatic injury in childhood, it may be so painful for them they must start putting Band-Aids on it, which distorts their sense of reality because they see the world differently. They start building the rest of their lives on a foundation that has a cornerstone ready to crumble.

I think we, as humans, can experience something like "soul lesions." This sounds pretty metaphysical, but we do know our whole being is an energy system and the trauma can be stored in what is known as the "muscle memory."

When the terms "soul lesions" and "muscle memory" were first introduced to me, another new door to healing opened for me. This topic is significant enough to be its own book and we won't go into more detail about it here, but I wanted to keep the introduction to the topic in here so readers who are interested in doing so may research this more on an individual basis.

Major Threat to Recovery

Treatment fatigue can be a major threat to a patient's recovery. A patient's condition is multifaceted. They have many different symptoms, and have been offered many different theories and ideas about those symptoms. Most patients have considered numerous treatment options and probably have experienced too many negative outcomes. This process can also lead to post-traumatic stress and anxiety, which we have covered elsewhere in the book.

The simplest forms of this can manifest as a frustration with the number of treatments and a loss of will to continue with the various recommended treatments. It can also manifest itself in much more severe forms.

Treatment fatigue can become a form of learned helplessness. One keeps trying without success; therefore, one is conditioned to believe that trying does not lead to success. So patients learn to stop trying and give up.

Why It Happens

One of the problems commonly encountered is when a patient develops a frustration with an approach to treatment. Even when they may be on the right track, they may often suddenly bail out of treatment by stopping all of their medications unilaterally without discussing the matter with their practitioner. If they were more open about their frustration with the practitioner, then the practitioner might be able to help them come in for a soft landing instead of a hard landing.

Sometimes, the reasons can be financial or philosophical. Sometimes, the patient is burned out on taking so many pills every day. Whatever the reason, it is critical to discuss them with the practitioner to find an appropriate alternative plan. It is always better to have a conversation with the practitioner, letting them know how you really feel, than to bail out and leave without explanation.

In the worst case scenario, a patient can be in the middle of an important treatment, bail out of the treatment and end up having a full relapse along with a greatly increased risk for developing antibiotic resistance because the germs were only partially treated and later can grow back.

Sometimes these microbes can grow back and induce a more intense host response after an episode like that. There are good medical reasons for not stopping in the middle of the course of treatment and that is true for any antibiotic regimen for any condition.

After a Long Course of Treatment

The most severe form of treatment fatigue will typically happen after a patient has been on a very long, frustrating and unsuccessful course of treatment. They might in their own mind have said, "I'm going to give this one more shot with so-and-so practitioner; if it doesn't work within 3.5 months I'm going to call it quits." They pre-program themselves to try it one more time with a certain unrealistic time frame and symptom response expectation; and if the target is not met they then justify it as a reason to bail out of the entire program. This kind of patient may ultimately not recover at all or continue to be sick for years longer.

There are many different ways of looking at this particular situation but there may be a subconscious reason the patient holds to not want to pursue a treatment even when they think it could be successful. Readiness is everything. Or depression may play a role.

Psychological Drivers

There are a variety of potential psychological drivers. For some patients, familiarity with an undesirable situation is less anxiety-provoking for them than unfamiliarity with a potentially better situation. This is an issue with change of many different kinds of behavior. Many books have been written on change management. It's also the basis for why many people endure abusive relationships.

For some, the familiar is more comforting than the potentially unfamiliar and unknown outcome. Ironically, I do think in some patients' cases, full recovery could present them with a set of options they are not ready to handle such as a return to a previously stressful role at work or at home.

After a chronic illness, most people don't want to go back to living the same way; sometimes it translates to a job or career change. It can translate to a change of lifestyle, of relationships, attachments, detachment, separations, divorce, etc. Sometimes, conversely, the healing cannot occur until the bad relationship the person is in actually ends.

We have seen a number of cases where separation or divorce began as the patient began to improve and feel well enough to realize: a) the situation they were in, and b) what they needed to do about it.

Reviewing What Does Work

It is helpful to review at each appointment not only what the problems are, but what problems have been solved; even if it is to touch on it very briefly so we can inventory and track what is and is not improving. This also helps direct the treatment in a more specific, successful way if you can discern and remember what the treatment actually did work on.

More time is spent for obvious reasons to talk about what is not working but time-and-time again, when I go through the list of

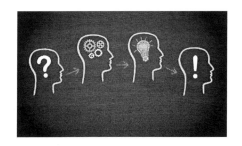

symptoms the patient initially provided, I can find many different completely resolved symptoms. When asked specifically about a symptom that was an issue at the beginning, a patient will say, "Oh yeah, that's all gone." They dismiss the wonderfulness of, the magnanimity of the fact that it is gone and then go on to focus on the issues at hand. Patients often do not realize they are improving.

As a patient improves, everyone around them may see improvement and their practitioner may see improvement. But as long as the patient is feeling badly, they are not going to necessarily be able to see a trend of emerging from the badness. The worse you feel, the smaller your world becomes.

It can be very, very difficult for a patient to develop and maintain a long-term perspective of their overall trend. Often, only when they are mostly out of it they can look back and say, "Yeah that was really bad and now I am out of it!" It may even be a normal, healthy trend for despondency yielding to frustration as a patient heals.

The treatment fatigue issue needs to be regularly considered by the patient and the practitioner together. Ideally, it would be a brief component of every appointment. It's important to get some sense from the patient at every appointment as to what extent they are on board with the process, how well it fits their situation and their mental receptiveness to the current recommended treatment. There is often a reasonable alternative approach available.

Sharon's Experiences with Treatment Fatigue

I was VERY lucky when I started with Dr. Mozayeni. I had not already been in treatment with numerous physicians. I didn't know what to expect. I knew I had felt horrible for years for various conditions; not realizing it was really all one disease.

When I started *Bartonella* treatment, I had no idea of the complexity of the disease or of the healing process. My ignorance allowed me to take things a month at a time. I wasn't looking six or twelve months down the road. I did what I needed to do until the next appointment. I didn't have a deadline. I didn't have any expectation of how much better to feel. I wanted to heal. Dr. Mozayeni told me from the start that in some ways I would feel worse before I felt better, so I didn't feel misled.

My treatment fatigue manifested a few times during treatment. First, and most commonly, I believe, was frustration over the number of pills I had to ingest on daily basis. I started out at 40 pills daily, at 8 different times of the day. It was a gargantuan task to organize and execute. It took me months to develop a workable system. The fatigue abated when I started to feel better, ever so slightly. I had a positive result for my efforts, so I had impetus for continuing.

My next incident of treatment fatigue occurred during the Hyperbaric Oxygen Therapy (HBOT) treatment to reduce inflammation (not as an anti-microbial). This process completely removed me from my co-workers and my friends. I was used to being with them on a daily basis. I felt extremely isolated, alone.

It was a difficult time for me (and my family). Later, after the treatment was complete, I noticed improved cognitive processing and the inflammation had subsided in parts of my body, thus reducing my overall pain levels. Again, the net gain has been significant, but man, it was tough getting there.

Treatment fatigue hit me again when I had to take other specific medications. The responses are so specific to each patient.

I came into Dr. Mozayeni's office and said, "Sorry, no can do this treatment..." I also got candida at that point. So, we compromised. We agreed together on the plan. I went off ALL antibiotic meds for a month, got rid of the candida, and psychologically took a break from treatment. I still took all my other prescription meds and supplements.

When I returned a month later, I was ready to start again. The first few doses were again horrible. So, I went back.

"I can't do this. It makes me too sick," I complained.

"How do you feel a few days after the doses?" he asked.

"Better."

"So, is the drug kicking ass then making you better or just making you sicker?" he queried.

"It's kicking ass and giving me a hell of a herx, but yes, it's working, not just making me sick," I said.

We agreed the drug was working. He got my buy-in into the healing process. I knew I needed to continue taking the med if I was going to heal. I had to figure out a way to get the drug in me but in a way I could tolerate. We talked and agreed how to move forward. Was it ideal for the protocol? No. Did I have to be on the drug longer? Yes. But the tradeoff was worth it to me so I wasn't so sick when I did take it.

The key here: when I felt the fatigue, I communicated it to Dr. Mozayeni. Often times, on my monthly Status Update, I would write, "I need to hear you aren't going to give up on me; that my case is not so frustrating or complex that you are going to stop wanting to treat me. I need to hear the confidence in your voice that I am on the path of healing."

Dr. Mozayeni has seen the gamut of chronically ill patients. He knew what was coming for me. He helped me stay focused on the end goal. Because I could maintain open communication lines with him, we made an excellent team and kept the treatment fatigue to a minimum.

SHARON

Some of my worst moments were before I was correctly diagnosed. I wanted to include them to give the reader validation for some of their own experiences and a realistic view of the treatment process to show that it waxes and wanes, but can eventually lead to healing.

Finished

"I'm done," Jeff stated flatly. "I've had it. I can't take it anymore. She has been sick for 20 years. I can't do this anymore." We were sitting in the marriage counselor's office. I remember feeling a stabbing pain in my gut. I had trouble hearing anything else out of his mouth. It was basically spew anyway. Angry spew.

We had been in marriage counseling off and on for years. Our therapist knew us well. But this was a place we had never gone before. I wanted none of it. I wondered what happened to the "in sickness and in health" part of the vows. Jeff reminded me I had been well for only two of our twenty years together; the first two. I think he thought I was making it all up. So did I really want to stay married to a man who didn't believe I was truly ill? It was an awful session filled with anger, resentment, fear, and complete sadness.

We were lucky. A couple of months later, I was on the right trail to diagnosis and healing. When Jeff finally heard a valid diagnosis, I think he decided to stick it out. Jeff tells his viewpoint of this moment elsewhere in this book.

Leaving

I don't remember at what point in the disease process this discussion occurred or what brought us together outside on our front porch on a sunny spring afternoon. The only snippet of the conversation I remember is when Jeff said, "So, if I am so hard to live with and so angry all the time, why are you staying with me?" His face was red, anger seething from his pores.

"Because I love you," I calmly and softly replied. And I meant it. "This anger isn't you. I don't know what it is or why it's there, but it's not you. So I am willing to wait and work through this together." Jeff shook his head and stormed off.

What we didn't know then, was that Jeff was experiencing what is called 'Lyme rage,' fits of anger that rise up and catapult the patient into raging behavior with no obvious cause and usually a quick conclusion. But what is said and done in the midst of that rage can be extremely damaging to a family and the relationships in that family.

The most amazing part of the healing process came four months into the treatment protocol; Jeff's rage completely disappeared.

Writing a Check

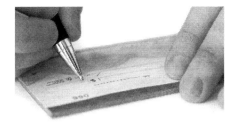

It was September 11th, 2008. I had attended a local memorial service that morning. I knew the date was important. But when I stood in my driveway to write a check, I could not remember the date. I couldn't even figure out what month it was. I was looking around the yard, searching for clues of at least what season we were in. My cat came around the corner of the garage and the only name I could pull up was a cat from my early childhood. I thought I was developing Alzheimer's.

Simple Things

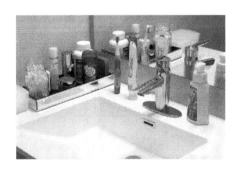

Sometimes, it's as simple as walking into the bathroom, picking up my toothbrush, looking at the bathroom counter, and not being able to tell which container is the tube of toothpaste. I had facial cleanser, eye make up remover, hair softener, and toothpaste sitting on the counter. I couldn't tell which one went on my toothbrush.

Incontinence

Incontinence is the final symptom I developed that got me 'beyond desperate' to find a cause of my symptoms. Utter defeat is the only way I can describe what I felt each time I lost control. It was the ultimate sign that at age 46, I had no control over my body.

Pets

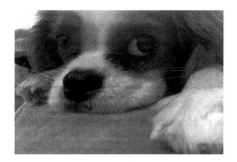

During treatment, one of our beloved dogs died of old age. Jeff drove me three hours each way to find Riley, a sweet, six month old Cavalier King Charles Spaniel puppy. Riley and I bonded - really bonded. I had never loved a dog as much I loved Riley. Less than a year later, Riley broke through our electric fence and was killed by a hit and run driver on our street.

Riley's sudden, horrific, tragic death devastated me. It ripped Jeff and me apart for a while. I had to find a way out of that grief to restart the healing process. At Dr. Mozayeni's suggestion, we went back to Riley's breeder and brought Lola and Rowdy home within the month. Puppies help rejuvenate the healing process.

Misreading the Label

While Jeff's and my treatments were staggered, there were times when we were on the same medications. And sometimes those meds were the same dosage, and sometimes not.

On one evening, Jeff and I took our meds at the kitchen counter and then proceeded to bed.

When I awakened the next morning, I couldn't speak. And I was hallucinating. Jeff thought I was having a stroke. I knew in my head what I wanted to say, but my words were completely garbled.

Two days later, we realized I had misread my prescription bottle. I took what should have been a lethal overdose of the medication. Miraculously, yes, miraculously, I survived and experienced no major organ damage. I lost the color in my vision for six days afterwards and then everything returned to normal.

When in treatment, patients can take anywhere between 30-70 pills daily (including supplements). If we don't read the bottles correctly, we can do much more damage than good.

Many of my worst "moments" weren't really moments. They were often a culmination of moments.

Getting Up

At the time I found out I had *Bartonella*, getting out of bed was agonizing. In my dreams, I could move, walk, run, and even fly. And even the first moments of awakening were delightful. But when I tried to move any muscle, reality would slap me awake, reminding me that the mere task of getting up and out of bed was still another 20-25 minutes away. My body felt heavy as concrete and as stiff as rebar. I had to spend the next period of time moving my joints in circles, loosening the ligaments. Eventually, I could move enough to get myself out of bed and to the bathroom.

Staying Up – Dysautonomia (Autonomic Nervous System Dysfunction)

It was January; Macy's was having a 70% off sale in the kitchen department. We needed a new skillet. I remember wearing a winter coat and Jeff was with me. We stood in the check out line with four people in line ahead of us. I was fine. And then I wasn't.

I broke into a cold sweat. My knees weakened. Suddenly, I needed a bathroom. IMMEDIATELY. Jeff led me to the bathroom and while I recovered, he bought and paid for the skillet. Ten minutes later, I was soaked in sweat, carrying my coat on my arm out of the bathroom, and tired. But I could stand and was no longer in pain. As fast as these episodes appeared, they would disappear with no rhyme or reason. They seemed to occur almost always as I was standing in line, or talking with a friend in a public place, whether it was Macy's or Safeway.

My mantra had become

> **"just because I could stand for the past five minutes does not mean I can stand for another minute."**

Other patients have shared similar stories regarding Postural Orthostasis Tachycardia Syndrome (POTS), which can be the result of vascular flow issues in the brain stem as well as vascular flow issues to the rest of the nervous system, such as the autonomic nervous system that regulates the tone of the blood vessels and the heart rate and the blood pressure.

Falling Down

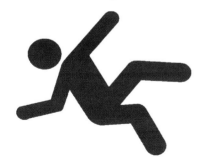

Because of my peripheral neuropathy, I don't always know where my feet are, literally. I don't always pick them up enough to clear my step, causing me to trip and fall. I have fallen and shattered my foot, spending seven weeks in bed in a cast with my leg elevated above my heart. I have sprained my ankles, knees and wrists.

I still fall occasionally and bang myself up. Nothing serious, but it knocks me out of my daily schedule for a week. It still takes me longer to recover from anything than most individuals. My fear of falling is sometimes immobilizing. I don't go out at night; I don't park in dark areas. And I am ALWAYS looking down at where I am walking to make sure I don't misstep.

Executive Functioning

For the last two years before I was properly diagnosed, I was completely unable to create an annual company budget. Too many days, I sat at my desk, completely paralyzed by the piles in front of me, unable to sort or prioritize any of the papers. My email inbox reached into the hundreds. What had come easily for me a few years prior had become impossible to even comprehend.

When creating the annual budget, reviewing the monthly company Profit and Loss, and paying bills was simply another task to check off, I knew the healing was happening.

Surgery

In June of 2009, my back pain had become so intense, I went to a spine specialist. An MRI later, I found out I had a lipoma. Next trips were to the neurosurgeon and back surgeon. One wanted to operate within six weeks; the other said he wasn't really sure if the lipoma was causing my back pain, but he wasn't sure what might be the cause instead.

I walked out of the last physician's office with a tiny voice inside of me saying, "This isn't the cause; keep looking." That message eventually led me within a couple of months to the Lupus test and then the right Lyme test.

All Made Up

I was allowed to wear make up as a teen. I rarely went without it. That lasted decades. Within months of starting into treatment, I stopped wearing make up entirely simply because I was too fatigued to put it on in the morning.

In southern culture, a woman isn't dressed if she doesn't have makeup applied. She is not 'presentable.' So, for me, to go without makeup was a MAJOR step. I was uncomfortable with the public and friends seeing me without it, but my fatigue was insurmountable and trumped that uncomfortableness.

For years, I went without makeup. Wanting to wear makeup again was a sign healing was happening for me. When I started wearing it regularly, but not religiously, I knew I was healing.

Break Time

It sounds ridiculous to many, until you live the moment when taking a shower is so exhausting it requires a 30 minute rest period afterwards. That's what happened to me. The fatigue was insurmountable. Between stiffness, joint pain, and fatigue, it was taking me two hours to get ready for work in the morning and that was with no makeup and putting on a pair of jeans and a t-shirt. I still don't understand why taking a shower can cause so much fatigue, but it seems to be common among Lyme patients to have to rest after bathing.

Stairs

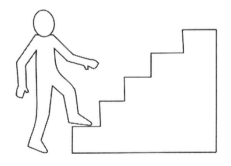

I stopped climbing stairs more than a year before I was properly diagnosed. Knee pain and weakness forbade me. If I had no alternative, I had to rest at every landing. I look like an 80 year-old when approaching even four steps at an office building. It is embarrassing and frustrating, but the pain incurred is too debilitating for me to be willing to take the stairs if there is any alternative. It is embarrassing not to be able to walk a flight of steps. But it is more embarrassing to have my husband or son literally help me up or down the steps while my knees crackle, pop, and sometimes completely give out.

Insomnia

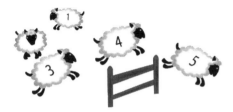

I suffered from insomnia for decades, completely unaware it had to do with my cortisol levels. Chronic infection had switched my adrenals into working at a crisis level on a constant basis. While most people's cortisol levels are at the lowest at night, that's precisely when mine would peak, forcing me into wakefulness that lasted until 2 or 4 am.

I crawled into bed at 10 pm, praying for sleep to take me, and then finally getting up before midnight, going into the guest room to get online, working, whatever my brain could handle for the next few hours.

Awakening at 6 am was treacherous. It didn't matter if I napped or didn't nap during the day; it seemed impossible to change the pattern. It left me feeling exhausted and frustrated; almost drugged. I could not get myself going in the morning.

Simon Says

During treatment, the progress was slow; tedious, really. When the medication was working, my symptoms temporarily worsened and then slightly improved. It wasn't even "three steps forward, two steps back." It was more like three steps forward, 2.75 steps back. It was six months into treatment before I believed I would really get better.

Sensory Overload

Movie theaters and malls became a nightmare for me. The lights were too bright; the audio in the movies was deafening. Within minutes of entering the mall, I became agitated and overwhelmed and fatigued. I couldn't decide which movie to see or what size popcorn to buy.

Choosing clothes became impossible. I learned to shop online. In fact, I didn't go in the mall for two years after I started treatment. That doesn't seem as big a deal now, but in 2009, it was significant.

SECTION SIX

PSYCHOLOGICAL THERAPIES FOR HEALING

"The healthy, the strong individual, is the one who asks for help when he needs it. Whether he has an abscess on his knee or in his soul."

– RONA BARRETT

SHARON

Characteristics of PTSD

Post Traumatic Stress Disorder (PTSD) is a stand-alone chapter because Dr. Mozayeni and I believe this condition is a core issue of most patients' chronic illnesses that complicates recovery.

Classic PTSD can occur following the experience or witnessing of a life-threatening events such as

- military combat
- natural disasters
- terrorist incidents
- serious accidents, or
- physical or sexual assault in adult or childhood.

Most survivors of trauma return to normal given a little time. However, some people will have stress reactions that do not go away on their own, or may even get worse over time. These individuals may develop PTSD.

People who suffer from PTSD often relive the experience through nightmares and flashbacks, have difficulty sleeping, and feel detached or estranged, and these symptoms can be severe enough and last long enough to significantly impair the person's daily life.

People with PTSD experience three different kinds of symptoms.

1. The first set involves reliving the trauma in some way such as becoming upset when confronted with a traumatic reminder or thinking about the trauma when trying to do something else.

2. The second set of symptoms involves either avoiding places or people that are reminders of the trauma, isolating from other people, or feeling numb.

3. The third set of symptoms includes things such as feeling on guard, irritable, or startling easily.

PTSD is marked by clear biological changes as well as psychological symptoms. People with PTSD often may develop additional disorders such as depression, substance abuse, problems of memory and cognition, and other problems of physical and mental health. PTSD is also associated with impairment of the person's ability to function in social or family life.

How PTSD Influences Treatment

The following contains excerpts from a conversation Dr. Mozayeni and I had on a Friday morning.

DR. MOZAYENI

The issue of post-traumatic stress disorder comes up often, but it is especially problematic in patients with chronic illness at the beginning and at the end of the treatment. I think it carries over into the process of treatment and makes it very hard sometimes for the patient to follow through with a regimen because it is hard to have faith in a process when you have had so many past negative experiences and you don't have faith in you pathway of care.

If not full-blown PTSD, patients at least present with a reasonable level of anxiety given what they have been through and this makes them hyper-vigilant about any other treatment they might consider.

This has profound, deep significance for both the patient and the practitioner. There is <u>no</u> way restorative therapy can start, and the patient can heal, and have a return to normal activity, if post-traumatic stress is complicating the process. For that matter, PTSD can actually completely prevent the process of healing and often causes the patient to be unable to follow **any** medical advice.

PTSD can affect the patient in three phases:

1. how they interact with us while we are interviewing them to qualify them to be a new patient.
2. how it affects them during treatment, and
3. how it affects their recovery and return to "normal activity."

In the beginning phase, they often will call a practitioner based on the reference of a friend, patient or someone they know on-line or even less commonly another practitioner. Depending on how much the referring individual said to them, they will call or come in with varying levels of concern and skepticism.

Most patients, when they initially arrive, are often so sick and have been sick for so long they cannot think clearly. This can be because of their anxiety and/or their illness causing cognitive impairment. They experience general anxiety and hyper-vigilance. That is not necessarily post-traumatic stress but it can be; they are in a survival mode where they are extremely anxious. The anxiety can block their rational thought.

Recently, I saw a patient who after a few years was so much better and was thanking me. I told her that when I first met her it seemed like she was in the middle of a five-alarm fire and she couldn't get herself calm enough to escape. She was fundamentally a smart person with severe disease-related anxiety. She was now thanking me with teary eyes. She is a totally different person now than when I first met her.

Responding to the Patient's Psychiatric Needs

The challenge for the clinician, especially for the internist, is to respond to psychiatric symptoms the way a psychiatrist might be able to do in a more objective detached way. The internist is more likely to label the patient and want to avoid them, dismiss them from the practice if they find they can't work with them early on rather than to recognize it is the patient's anxiety stemming from whatever they have been through and the situation they are in so that they can be calmed down, relaxed, and able to proceed with treatment.

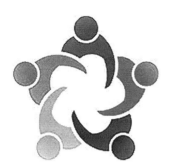

This is multidisciplinary. This is to have a team approach wit. psychiatrist, or psychotherapist conjunction with the internist. While t managing the patient's emotions, the in __st can be the engineer working out logistically what needs to be done to solve the puzzle from a biochemical, immunological, and metabolic point of view.

In the early phases of treatment the patient needs to understand they are starting a journey. Most journeys are somewhat anxiety-provoking because they are somewhat unpredictable - there are bumps in the road and turbulence in the atmosphere that you have to endure as you travel to your destination. Someone who is already compromised is being asked to shift out of whatever homeostasis or balance they have achieved. You are asking them to change that. There will be aspects of their illness that will improve while there are aspects of their illness that will worsen before they get better.

It can take four-to-six months or more and many anxiety-driven phone calls often requiring calm and compassionate answers of their repetitive questions. Repetitive questions may be indications of cognitive impairment and anxiety, which go hand-in-hand. A patient's high adrenaline state can severely impair short-term memory. It is a known fact:

learning does not occur well or at all

in someone in a high-adrenaline state.

As we try to restore the patient, we are also disrupting their routine when asking them to follow a new routine. Here, they need to call upon their faith in the process and do what is the hardest thing to do: **surrender to the process**. But to do that, they have to have the **trust the process.** If they have post-traumatic stress from past experiences with other physicians and practitioners who were not able to help them, the patients cannot have trust in that process until they get better and it is proven to them the practitioner should have that trust.

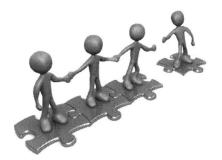

This period of time is really one of the most difficult periods in treatment because it is as difficult for the staff of our practice as it is for the patient. Since some of our staff members weren't trained to be mental health workers they sometimes have an emotional response to a patient rather than a clinical, analytical response to that patient.

There's an important point here to be made which is with a patient who is seeing a psychiatrist: usually there is only the psychiatrist and maybe one other staff member in a very small office, often in a home office setting. Whereas when the patient is working with an Internal Medicine practice there are multiple other patients and staff, so the odds of negative encounters increases. There are several staff members and there is potentially less one-on-one time for the patient with the clinician.

That is operationally one of the key distinguishing features of these two different worlds of internal medicine and psychiatry. Over time we try to blend together and bring in traits that psychiatrists have been trained to have and the skills they have developed; to bring those into Internal Medicine to be able to better manage the patient's mental health as we take them through an Internal Medicine fix for their systemic illness that relates so tightly to their mental health.

Effect of PTSD on Treatment

What about post-traumatic stress in the course of treatment? We covered what PTSD looks like in the first six months of treatment. Later on during the treatment there will be many phases, many smaller versions of what was seen during that initial six-month period. Potentially with any new therapy, or change in regimen, any major transition point where a treatment protocol is substantially altered or terminated based on a new test result, could result in another crisis.

Every one of these changes of treatment and new diagnostic information has the potential to create a sort of crisis for the patient.

I think most clinicians usually don't hear from the patient exactly how big each of these steps may be.

It is important to continually strive to improve the process. One of the things that will do the most to lower people's anxiety about these steps is to have ever better data collected demonstrating the validity and risks of whatever decisions are being made. We need better data support driving real-time decisions so that we can take the angst out of the decision on the part of the patient and the practitioner.

Importance of PTSD Therapy for Complete Healing

I also think it is critical for the patient to be in some kind of counseling or psychotherapy for PTSD throughout treatment. PTSD can be brought on by their experiences in the medical system, but it can also be caused by other experiences in their life that have nothing to do with medicine. But the PTSD nevertheless significantly impacts the treatment process.

The patient needs to have someone to go to when a big change occurs in the treatment protocol to help deal with those changes and the feelings they bring up. Though outwardly they may not appear to be connected, they often are and their fears need to be addressed by a trained professional.

Fears and concerns cross-react, synergize, and amplify one another.

I think the absolute best possible scenario for managing someone with a chronic illness is when they jointly see their internist, who is problem-solving the complexity of their case, while concurrently, they are in counseling with various kinds of mental health professionals. The mental health aspect should be managed by a trained psychiatrist familiar with the internal medicine protocols and PTSD therapy.

I think a lot of damage can be done if the therapist has not been trained as a mental health professional in PTSD, especially with chronic illness.

We are always improving our protocols. We are trying to find and set up a whole program wherein people who are experts in PTSD can talk to patients and routinely and help them move through and see the distinction among the different sources of their stress so a past traumatic event from something else completely unrelated to medicine doesn't interfere with their medical progress. This is critical to patients' healing. It's a very important point.

In the last phase of treatment, when you have a patient who is mostly well and has the ability now to start thinking about where they are going and how their life will look after the illness, there is a whole new kind of PTSD.

Patient Transformation

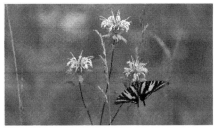

©JOE KELLY

The other problem faced by patients in this situation is that they have been transformed by their illness. Their awareness of medicine has changed. They have an awareness of the potential for chronic infections to affect their lives. They have a higher level of spiritual awareness given the trials and tribulations they have been through and the faith they have had to bring forward in order to sustain the process of getting well.

These individuals are changed by their illness experience. They have undergone a lot of involuntary growth. Their bodies are weary from exposure to meds, chemicals and supplements. They have a significant treatment fatigue related to the fact that they have had to take so much medicine, do so many things for their therapy for so long. All of that spells for a deep interest and desire **not** to go back to doing what they were doing before.

It is not necessarily about not going back to the relationships they had before. Some of them, in the course of this illness, have separated from some old relationships, which ironically, in almost every case I have seen where that has happened, has actually accelerated their healing. This should be good news. It could be really good news for someone who is worried about a relationship ending, say with a spouse.

More than anything, patients crave being able to take what they have learned and transcend where they were and do something better, to be someone better, to help others. They usually want to transition to having the highest possible altruism.

A lot of the patients who go through this, whatever field of life they are in, they come out of this thing saying, "All I want to do is help people." Suddenly, they see all that is moot and insignificant. Their primary objective becomes wanting to heal others and increase their ability to love others and to heal them through love. It's spiritually transformational.

Patient as Healer

The patient also has a role in a sense as a healer, for the medical staff and the practitioner. Everyone is, at some level, naturally a healer and who wants to help. When a medical team is doing everything it can, working hard to take care of someone, the team gets tremendous fulfillment from a patient's successful healing. When the patient follows the treatment plan, has some success, has a healthy working relationship with those involved with the treatment; *that* is **hugely** satisfying for the medical team taking care of them. It is what keeps most practitioners in this kind of practice.

The practitioners can be feeling burnt out, stressed, and intimidated by guidelines, laws, regulations, reimbursement, and malpractice.

The patient, especially when ill, can be challenged with being polite, conscientious, and ethical; it can also be challenging not to make unreasonable demands or false accusations.

The medical team needs to follow these guidelines as well, keeping in mind that the patient may react badly at times due to the anxiety and frustrations they are experiencing. If everyone maintains civility, the path to healing is much simpler.

SHARON

When I finished my *Bartonella* treatment, I brought in a dozen cupcakes for the staff to enjoy. I wanted to mark the day with something, and cupcakes were the fad. The staff sees us at our worst, but they don't always see the positive markers. I liked being able to show my appreciation for their compassion and kindness.

Living with Lyme can be exhausting for the patient and families. But it can also be exhausting for the medical staff. One of my tools for healing was to reach out to others, whether to offer support, or sometimes, or express gratitude for those around me who were helping me heal. I brought in samples of the green smoothies I had been drinking and sugar free desserts I was trying. Sometimes I wanted them to commiserate with me on this journey, but mostly I wanted them to feel a part of my healing process.

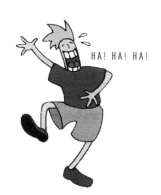

HA! HA! HA!

Laughter and hope are key elements to my healing, but they are also key elements to a healthy staff. And the laughter between the two is essential, encouraging a lighter spirit and a positive environment.

Transformation for Practitioners

Practitioners are also transformed. Once you start treating people with these conditions, particularly if you have been really successful at it, it changes you. It changes how you look at **everything**.

It's transforming the same way I think patients are transformed. It's a spiritual experience. You see multiple patients going through multiple spiritual experiences in their recovery. There is no way you cannot have a similar transformation to what the patients have. You cannot heal unless you care, and if you care, it can be emotionally exhausting.

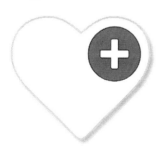

In my case it was about trying to process the emotionality of it all. It reached a point where if I continued to pursue it analytically, it was too stressful. There was all this analytical headwork but there was none of the benefit that you get out of working from the heart.

I needed to find a way to process the questions in a way that would not only make it easier but actually enable me to deal with the most difficult situations in a way that wasn't stressful. I can only describe it in the most general way right now, as I am still in the midst of the transformation.

SHARON

I wonder what it is like for you. The patients see their own miracle of healing but you potentially see multiple healing miracles each day. I know you still see a lot of sick people, but you do see more of the healing than say the average patient does because they only see their own.

DR. MOZAYENI

I've described the process to patients as my being there to show them the ladder to recovery, every rung on the ladder, one rung at a time. Because I have helped people up multiple ladders I know they can do it. I know how it's done because I know what the rungs look like.

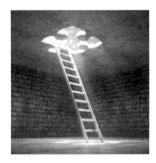

You get that perspective, but on a day-to-day basis you might get one patient with a big breakthrough. The majority of interactions you have each day are arduous. It is real work to get to the point where you have that big breakthrough one person at a time.

Staying spiritually and energetically clear and centered is extremely important because you are dealing with people who are constantly pulling energy from you - they are trying to center themselves.

Like a lifeguard going out to a drowning victim, you've got to be there and help but you've got to know when to kind of pull back slightly so you don't get pulled down. A drowning victim will literally try to stand on your head and will drown you in the process. It's one of the first things they teach lifeguards: how to get out of those grips.

Eye Movement Desensitization and Reprocessing (EMDR) and Somatic Experiencing (SE)

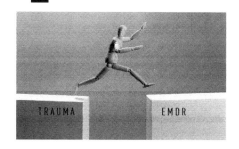

An important element of EMDR and SE therapies is for the patient to develop a deep awareness of their body; to become tuned in with their body's physical responses. As a chronically ill patient with chronic pain, I had spent years trying to ignore the messages my body sent to me; a very common characteristic of PTSD patients.

This therapy was asking me to pay close attention to <u>every</u>thing my body did and messaged to me whenever I thought about or emotionally experienced things. This single task took me a very long time to develop. It was not easy. It sounded simple.

"What is your body feeling right now as we talk about this?" the therapist asked.

"I feel upset and frightened," I responded.

"But what is your body feeling? Are any muscles tense? What is your breathing like?" she queried.

I had to break my body down into sections and run a mental scan to see what it was my body was feeling. It was a slow, laborious process for me. But it was essential to create a positive therapeutic effect.

I could then find relationships between events that caused me emotional stress or difficulty and how it translated to my body's reaction. By finding the correlation, I could then work on lowering my body's stress reaction and creating opportunities for it to become a healing agent.

EMDR

EMDR therapy was developed by Francine Shapiro, Ph.D. in 1987. It is used for individuals who have experienced severe trauma that remains unresolved. According to Shapiro, when a traumatic or distressing experience occurs, it may overwhelm normal cognitive and neurological coping mechanisms. The memory and associated stimuli are inadequately processed and stored in an isolated memory network.

The goal of EMDR therapy is to process the distressing memories, reducing their lingering effects and allowing patients to develop more adaptive coping mechanisms. This is done in an eight-step protocol that includes having clients recall distressing images while receiving one of several types of bilateral sensory input, including side-to-side eye movements.

Shapiro noticed that certain eye movements appeared to reduce the intensity of disturbing thoughts. She conducted a scientific study in 1989. The success rate of that first study using trauma victims was posted in the Journal of Traumatic Stress. Shapiro noted that, when she was experiencing a disturbing thought, her eyes were involuntarily moving rapidly. She noticed further that, when she brought her eye movements under voluntary control while thinking a traumatic thought, anxiety was reduced.

Shapiro developed EMDR therapy for post-traumatic stress disorder. In that 1989 study, she speculated that traumatic events "upset the excitatory/inhibitory balance in the brain, causing a pathological change in the neural elements." EMDR is now recommended as an effective treatment for emotional trauma in the *Practice Guidelines* of the American Psychiatric Association.

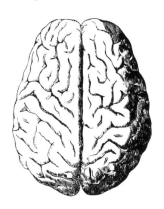

Numerous patients have successfully used EMDR as part of their healing whether it involves dealing with family of origin issues, a single traumatic event, or otherwise. Many stated that while they can't efficiently describe HOW it works, they do know it works well and it works quickly. Also noted was the positive aspect of not having to use "talk therapy" to deal with a trauma. They didn't have to "dredge up the past" in order to start the healing process.

Somatic Experiencing

Somatic Experiencing (SE) is a form of therapy aimed at relieving and resolving the symptoms of post-traumatic stress disorder (PTSD) and other mental and physical trauma-related health problems by focusing on the client's perceived body sensations (or somatic experiences). It was introduced in Dr. Peter Levine's 1997 book *Waking the Tiger*.

In it, he discusses at length his observations of animals in the wild, and how they deal with and recover from life-threatening situations. According to Levine, the lower brain structures that regulate biological processes and maintain life become disorganized during traumatic experiences that are too severe for the lower brain structures and body to cope with. Most of the time, the disorganization is temporary or short term.

Not all individuals subject to a traumatic event are necessarily traumatized by it. Most of the time, people who are traumatized by an event return to healthy function. When traumatic symptoms do persist, it is often because the lower brain structures have not returned to their healthy function.

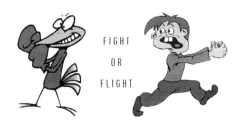

FIGHT OR FLIGHT

The impact of enduring traumatic stress in the body can leave it in a state of high arousal geared toward the basic survival responses of orienting, a sort of fight or flight response. The other basic survival response, freeze and dissociation, also has a high level of potential or actual arousal. This stress is common among chronically ill patients.

When the body and lower brain structures remain disorganized after a traumatic event, they have failed to regulate themselves back to health through the inherent self-regulatory mechanisms and processes that nature had provided. Such situations call for conscious interactive regulation by the higher brain structures and/ or the environment.

This can be compared to when you break a bone, it often cannot heal by itself. It is set in place and held in a cast from the outside for the healing to take place on its own on the inside through inherent biological processes involving interactions between the body and the brain structures.

The purpose of Somatic Experiencing is to use the brain's higher functioning structure to bring the lower functioning structure back into line; into the healthy functioning capacity. In SE, the patient is taught to break the cycle of being reminded of an event and responding to the event in a healthy fashion rather than the survival cycle it originally learned during the traumatic event.

Somatic Experiencing should be conducted only by licensed therapists thoroughly trained in the therapy.

While writing this book, I found my journal I was keeping during my recovery. These are some notes regarding EMDR and SE:

Two months into treatment

11/4/09 - Driving to EMDR, I have to traverse over a bridge. I try to speed up on bridges. My eyes dart back and forth, wondering if it will fall and I will be one of the victims of an unexpected bridge collapse.

Bridges are the transitional phrases in life. I'm not here or there. I am traveling from here to there. I am in between. I don't like being in between. I want that solid foundation beneath me.

This *Bartonella* has put me in a transition place for at least two years. I have to kill off the bacteria in stages, one by one. I can't skip, or go in circles, or I won't make it to the wellness stage.

When fear strikes, when my symptoms worse or intensify, the fear intrudes and imprisons the disease. My body goes in lock down mode. My spine becomes a rod of steel through which nothing can pass. It is trying to help the best way it knows how.

Since most of my symptoms are on the right, it tries to block the bacteria from moving to the left. But it also blocks the healing energy. It keeps my body out of balance and therefore unable to move correctly and eventually unable to heal.

I need a pendulum slowly moving back and forth, left and right. Quietly, patiently, the energy can move through the body. It's not a race; it's a marathon. I have to pace myself. I breathe in deeply, hold for a moment, exhale, allowing the energy to pass through me in every direction, allowing oxygen to move freely thru my muscles, tissues, tendons, and even bones. My right side keeps twitching. Then, my right foot relaxes. My right shoulder drops a bit, my chin lifts higher so I am no longer bowing my head.

My spine becomes my support, not my prison. Vertically, it strengthens and lengthens. Horizontally, I become a pass-through for all of my energy, allowing an even flow, side to side.

This is how the battle will be won. Inch by inch - with motion. I cannot give up; I cannot freeze. I need to keep the body and spirit moving. Don't get locked in, frozen or stuck.

Four months into treatment:

1/12/10 - The disconnect between body and brain can be standard in a society where we are constantly rushing from one place to another, literally and figuratively.

My list of To Dos doesn't incorporate rest time or even a self-check in time. It is go, gO, GO.

If the body isn't ready, the cortisol and adrenaline hormones kick in to keep the body moving while the brain continues pushing through the schedule and crossing items off the To Do list.

So when I sit in the therapist's office and she asks me how I'm feeling, I tend to use my brain as the reference point.

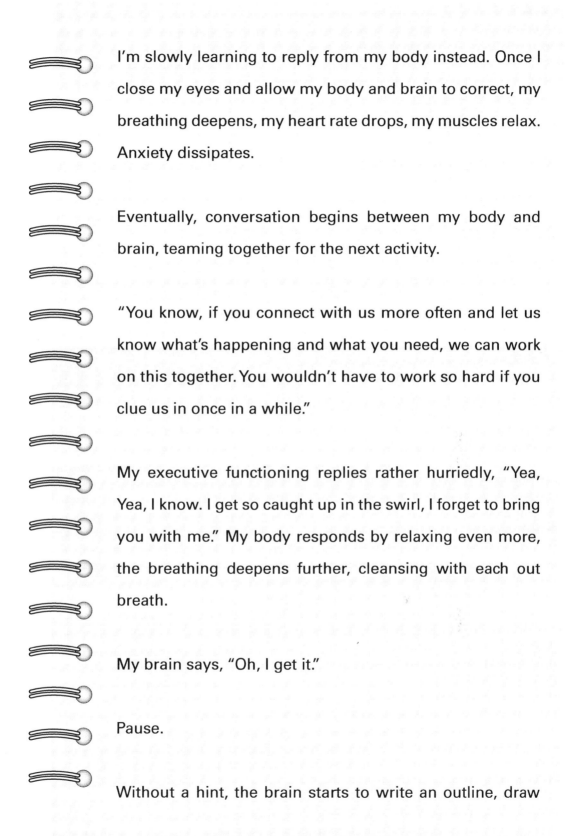

I'm slowly learning to reply from my body instead. Once I close my eyes and allow my body and brain to correct, my breathing deepens, my heart rate drops, my muscles relax. Anxiety dissipates.

Eventually, conversation begins between my body and brain, teaming together for the next activity.

"You know, if you connect with us more often and let us know what's happening and what you need, we can work on this together. You wouldn't have to work so hard if you clue us in once in a while."

My executive functioning replies rather hurriedly, "Yea, Yea, I know. I get so caught up in the swirl, I forget to bring you with me." My body responds by relaxing even more, the breathing deepens further, cleansing with each out breath.

My brain says, "Oh, I get it."

Pause.

Without a hint, the brain starts to write an outline, draw

pictures, presenting a book, telling the body what is coming soon. Today, my brain is telling me about the antibiotics I'm going to be starting in a few weeks. A calendar appears with the dates, a television shot of me sitting in Dr. Mozayeni's office, going thru the next check-up and talking about the weeks to come.

I see myself bringing a television into bedroom with a remote control, the house phone now has an extension sitting on my night stand. Fresh sheets on the bed. The blinds are closed. The house is quiet. Jammer, my cat, sleeps next to the heating pad under my back. His breathing is slower than mine.

My body remains calm and relaxed while it views all this. I envision the antibiotics permeating my body down to the cellular level, capturing the bacteria and demolishing them with one big gulp. My muscles remain relaxed.

For weeks, my body will be completely depleted of energy. It's important for me to rest at a restorative level and let this process happen.

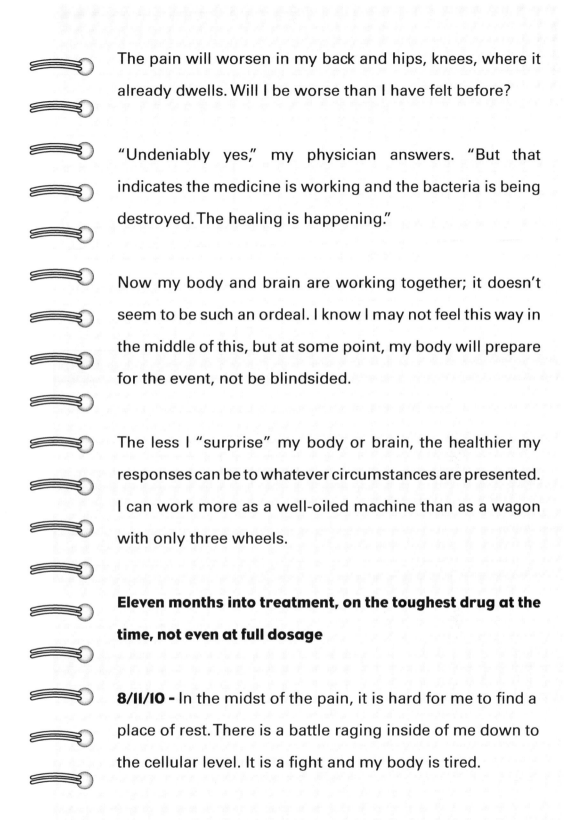

The pain will worsen in my back and hips, knees, where it already dwells. Will I be worse than I have felt before?

"Undeniably yes," my physician answers. "But that indicates the medicine is working and the bacteria is being destroyed. The healing is happening."

Now my body and brain are working together; it doesn't seem to be such an ordeal. I know I may not feel this way in the middle of this, but at some point, my body will prepare for the event, not be blindsided.

The less I "surprise" my body or brain, the healthier my responses can be to whatever circumstances are presented. I can work more as a well-oiled machine than as a wagon with only three wheels.

Eleven months into treatment, on the toughest drug at the time, not even at full dosage

8/11/10 - In the midst of the pain, it is hard for me to find a place of rest. There is a battle raging inside of me down to the cellular level. It is a fight and my body is tired.

EMDR and SE help me reconnect with a time when my body felt energized, well, able to move, vibrant. I connect to when I was five and seeing snow for the first time.

It's important that I do not go back to that time; rather I reconnect with it and bring it forward.

Our bodies do not know the concept of time.

Time exists in our brains only.

When I have been in pain for so long, it can be hard to remember a time when my body felt well. But when I do have the moment, <u>that</u> is what I need to reconnect with.

I need to bring _that_ moment to the present and keep it as my reservoir or oasis that I can dip into at any moment when I need to feel refreshed and rejuvenated.

Even if not physically, I can use it psychologically and emotionally. It is my remembering that my body will feel that way again.

PSYCHOLOGICAL THERAPIES AND SUPPORT

SHARON

I came to Dr. Mozayeni in 2009 so he could heal me. I had no idea the journey that lay ahead of me. I thought I just needed the right medications. While that part is true, I quickly discovered my healing needed to be three fold: physical, emotional/mental, and spiritual.

This does NOT mean that if you wish it hard enough, you will heal. Or if you don't think the right things, you cannot heal. That's *not* what this chapter is about.

Many chronically ill patients have some common characteristics even though we come from all walks of life. Many of us are intuitive, sensitive, "feelers." We can often "sense" something in others, get a "gut feeling," or feel the "energy" in a room. This may not account for all patients, but it does seem to fit a majority of the patients I have met. Other patients have shared with me similar findings.

The beginning of my healing required two things that had nothing to do with medication. It required acceptance and healing.

Acceptance

From childhood, I thought acceptance meant I condoned or approved of things; whatever had happened to me was ok by me. I couldn't do that. I spent so many years not accepting physicians' diagnoses,

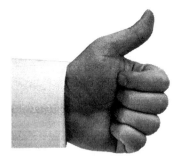

not accepting their treatments; refusing to give up. I paralleled acceptance with passivity and being docile.

Acceptance is an acknowledgement.

Accepting is not the same as giving permission. Accepting is not the same as liking or condoning or approving.

I can accept my circumstances, my life, people, and even events around me, *without* giving my approval or releasing my control over such. I don't have to like what is happening; I do need to accept that it indeed is happening.

Once I accepted what was happening to my body, I could plan accordingly.

For instance, some of my medications caused extreme fatigue. Instead of trying to "soldier on" with my normal schedule, I made a conscious decision not to leave the house after 5 pm on weeknights. On the weekends, I scheduled one activity for the entire two days. The rest of the time I allowed for resting. This was a significant change for me. But I realized an essential part of my healing could only happen is my body was rested and rejuvenated. Rest was the first step. If I wasn't rested, then my body had no energy left for healing.

Some individuals laughed at me for such major restrictions on my schedule. And a few were even annoyed. I ignored the snide remarks, knowing healing was my number one priority.

Acceptance is not giving permission, liking, condoning, or approving of something.

Acceptance is simply an acknowledgement of what exists.

Willingness

"Try drinking a tablespoon of apple cider vinegar before dinner."

Pause.

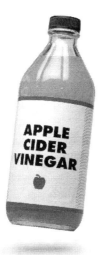

"Apple cider vinegar? Are you nuts?" I blurted out.

I think that was my third appointment with Dr. Mozayeni. I was completely unwilling to try his suggestion only because it sounded yucky.

Four months later, after developing yeast issues in my

body, I tried the apple cider vinegar. Then I started drinking it daily. And the yeast disappeared.

During another appointment in my first eight months of treatment, Dr. Mozayeni suggested I try green smoothies for some of my gut issues (diarrhea, bloating, pain).

"Next topic, because I am SO NOT DOING THAT," I emphatically stated. Three months later, I tried green smoothies out of desperation. And they worked. I found the type that worked for me and then I became a green smoothie "enthusiast."

Willingness.
If I found myself unwilling to try something,
I prayed for the "willingness to be willing."

This disease ravaged my body. Healing took time and a little trial and error. And some healing came from the most unexpected places – like a bottle of apple cider vinegar and in a Vitamix blender with spinach. In order to heal, I needed to remain aware and accept the possibilities.

Keeping these two characteristics in mind, let's move forward with some of the other activities and therapies that patients might find helpful.

Support Groups & Message Boards

One of the most common complaints from chronically ill patients is a sense of loneliness. If no one else in the family suffers from the same illness, there is no one close to compare notes with; no one to commiserate with.

The advancement of social media has given patients opportunities to connect and network with one another. Whereas the only choice a few years ago might have been a local support group that met once a month, now patients can hop online any time of day or night and connect with someone else with similar symptoms, treatment, and overall life situation.

Message boards are also helpful when searching for physicians or similar symptom sets. Social media like Facebook and Twitter offer immediate feedback and responses to patients' questions. Social media gives patients a place to bond, to connect, and to laugh WITH each other.

It is important to find others who are HEALING, and not STUCK in their illness. And by healing, I don't mean necessarily that they are getting physically better every day. It's important to find others who are as determined to heal as you are. Find the ones who continue moving forward. Find the ones who are constantly trying to live in the solution and not wallowing in the problem.

Meditation & Prayer

There are innumerable studies and surveys available indicating the benefits of prayer and meditation in relationship to healing and general health.

Three years after I started treatment, a friend offered me the opportunity to do a 21-day meditation challenge sponsored by Deepak Chopra and Oprah Winfrey. I had tried numerous meditation tapes and programs over the years and I didn't like any of them. I frankly didn't hold much hope for this 21-day challenge. But I knew the spiritual aspect was an important element to my healing.

Fortunately, for me, the 21-day challenge worked. I ended up finding some other meditation programs that Deepak Chopra had developed and now I am much more consistent in this practice.

That doesn't mean I meditate every day. It means I do it as often as I can and I know when I do meditate, my mind is quieter, my body is calmer, and my attitude is overall positive and moving in a forward direction.

I also practiced Transcendental Meditation™ and found it helpful.

Meditation often helps with sleep and anxiety disorders. I encourage patients to keep trying different meditation programs until you find something you like. Don't give up. Not all meditation programs are the same!

During treatment, I also attended a Centering Prayer retreat that offered a different type of meditation.

Meditation is not necessarily a spiritual or religious activity. It is simply a technique to quiet the mind, which can help facilitate healing on all levels. You can make meditation into what you need it to be. And when those needs change, meditation is very flexible.

Regardless of what I choose, I believe incorporating prayer and/or meditation is a key element to overall healing.

qEEG and Cranial Electrical Stimulation

I definitely don't always get the science of a device, but I know the qEEG saved me valuable time when I fell into a deep depression during treatment and needed medication quickly. I had tried MANY antidepressant medications over the years and the only one that had significantly helped had been taken off the market.

"Here, try this medication for six weeks and we'll see how it does for you." Those six-week intervals were nothing but sheer hell for me.

I did the qEEG and found one specific drug was really the only medication that would probably work for me. And it did. Beautifully.

DR. MOZAYENI

We are going to talk about brain waves, quantitative EEG, regular EEG, brain electrical patterns, electrical mapping and a device that uses electrical stimulation to help improve insomnia, anxiety, and depression. That device is called a Fisher Wallace Cranial Electrical Stimulator. You can read about it at www.fisherwallace.com.

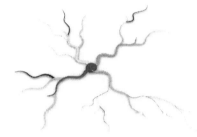

The brain, like any other organ, is fed by the vascular system and because the brain and the nerves are so intricate and do so many things, the brain and the nervous system become very sensitive detectors of any abnormality of vascular function and vascular flow. When one has small-vessel disease there can be neuropsychiatric symptoms including fatigue, emotional instability, memory issues, and so forth.

If a certain part of the brain is being affected at a particular moment by some piece of biofilm or very small clot traveling through the circulation or some inflammation in that vascular branch, that part of the brain's function will be more selectively affected at that moment.

This explains why people with small-vessel disease and chronic inflammation may have sudden episodes of mood changes or sudden episodes of forgetfulness or episodes of anxiety or lightheadedness, nausea, or even peripheral nerve symptoms.

There are parts of the brain stem that regulate blood pressure so if you have an instability to your blood pressure such as POTS (Postural Orthostasis Tachycardia Syndrome) which can be affected, it could be the result of vascular flow issues in the brain stem as well as vascular flow issues to the rest of the nervous system, such as the autonomic nervous system that regulates the tone of the blood vessels and the heart rate and the blood pressure.

The brain temporal lobes could also be affected, causing mood disturbances, visual processing and word finding. If the frontal lobes are affected, causing diminished neurotransmitter production, the result would be a compromise of will. If you have frontal lobe compromise you can have apathy, lethargy, or dis-inhibition and inappropriate behavior. If it affects the deeper structures of the thalamus, it can affect emotions and mood.

There are known vascular lesions that can cause sudden mood changes and tearfulness. Vascular lesions can also affect the perception of contrast by the part of the brain that sees, the occipital lobe. So visual acuity and contrast sensitivity are other examples of how vascular inflammation can compromise aspects of brain function.

In addition, parts of the brain can be affected in a way that causes narcolepsy. Potentially, any function of the brain can be affected by vascular compromise to that particular region of the brain.

Because of all of these interruptions in vascular flow one can have a multitude of different symptoms in the brain; and the brain, like any part of the body, actually has electrical activity.

Because it does, we can do an electroencephalogram, an EEG. We can also look at peripheral nerve and muscle conduction studies. That's an EMG/NCV, electromyogram and nerve conduction velocity study. Other parts of the body have electrical signals too.

When it comes to the brain, EEGs have been used for various reasons. It was first used to detect major bursts of electrical discharge that correlated with seizure disorders. In the early days of the technology the equipment was not as sensitive to the minor fluctuations and the lower voltage discharges. Over the years, advances in electronics have allowed manufacturers of EEG equipment to develop more sensitive methods of detecting and measuring the electrical current. With the advent of computational power they have now learned to use the electrical patterns to map the brain, and more recently, to correlate those maps with response to specific medications.

In the same way you might look into space with an infrared telescope or a radio telescope or look at gamma rays in the sky, one can also apply various filters and look at different frequencies of electrical patterns in the brain and then use computers to actually map out where those different signals and patterns are coming from in the different parts of the brain. All that can be done by simply applying some electrodes to the surface of the brain where we are measuring incredibly tiny voltages and learning to see an ever more amazing richness of detail in the electrical patterns.

One of the things you might see in someone who has had vascular injury or other injury to the brain is that they will have a dis-coordination of the brain wave patterns between and among the different parts of the brain. There are different waves that occur during sleep. Deep, slow brain waves known as delta waves begin to emerge during Stage 3 sleep. Stage 3 is a transitional period between light sleep and a very deep sleep. Some patients with brain injury from these illnesses will have those waves become more prominent when their eyes are open than when they are closed.

You might also see parts of the brain that have different kinds of signaling, or different frequencies, and that they are also mismatched. You can look at the brain mapping and if you see patterns that are inconsistent with normal, you now have electrical evidence that validates what the patient has been trying to tell you with regard to their symptoms.

In addition to those brain-mapping approaches, there is a methodology referred to as quantitative EEG. The quantitative EEG allows the brain wave patterns to be looked at from a bio-statistical point of view. We can use statistics and computational power to see present correlations or ratios.

We have the ability to look at flow dynamics, brain electrical patterns, and pixels on various scans (SPECT, PET, MRI scan); each of these provides a certain kind of information. None of these will be as good alone as they will in conjunction with everything else.

Ultimately one hopes that for some conditions and in at least some situations, this methodology of mapping out the brain's electrical patterns could then provide a short list of suggestions for mental health medication usage.

An electrical pattern might be documented on a quantitative EEG, then correlated with responsiveness to some antidepressant. It might also be used to correlate with improvement from certain stimulants like Adderall or Ritalin. Potentially these patterns could be used to better inform, or better yet, to prioritize what meds might be attempted first.

We don't want to rely on these 100%, especially because they are new. They are going to be controversial at first. We might find over time they do a better job of being able to sort out which medication is best used and to prioritize which ones are used to make this less of a random search for an effective medication. We hope through a variety of diagnostics and indices developed across a variety of different measurement techniques, not only electrical, that we can come up with a more rational and efficient framework for figuring out what meds would work if we have to use medications.

Potential Avenues of Treatment Using Electrical Patterns and Electrical Signals

The quantitative EEG is a diagnostic aid. Cranial Electrical Stimulation (CES) is a therapeutic device.

The very first uses of cranial electrical stimulation were extreme, used to take people out of major depression, so-called electroshock therapy. This continues to be used for severely depressed patients unresponsive to treatment.

CES devices are *not* electroshock therapy.

New CES devices that are used today are portable, hand-held. They are very comfortable to use, easy to wear. You can put it on and stick the small unit in your pocket or on your belt clip and go about doing your routine.

CES devices provide micro currents of electrical frequencies to the brain. The simplest method is to apply two wet sponges held by

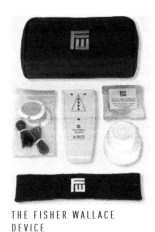

THE FISHER WALLACE
DEVICE

an elastic head strap. They are held in place right above and to the front of the ear. They are simple. The device has a volume knob that you can set to one of four settings. On lower settings it tends to be calming. It helps with anxiety and insomnia. On higher settings it tends to be stimulatory and can help with depression.

In a typical patient who might have been heavily medicated for all sorts of mood, anxiety, and thought disorders, under the close supervision of a psychiatrist, it may be possible to wean off medications while using the CES. Once the medications have been eliminated, a quantitative EEG can be done to help personalize the medication choice. But first, the cranial electrical stimulator could be applied to help with the symptoms of insomnia, anxiety, or depression. If it is ineffective, the newly chosen medication could be started.

This process outlined is definitely not for everyone and it would have to be done carefully under a psychiatrist's supervision but is an example of how these diagnostic techniques have the potential to change the neuropsychiatric aspects of these conditions.

The single biggest reason in my mind for trying not to use medications is because if you have an underlying cause of your symptoms identified such as a chronic infection, the neuropsychological manifestations may change and often improve rather quickly. Because it takes a long time to search for, find and stabilize the right psychiatric medications, the time frame for successful treatment of the neuropsychological manifestations is much longer than the time frame for the diagnosis and treatment for Lyme Disease and related infections.

A patient could end up being a moving target for the medication because the underlying disease process is being remediated or changed on a time scale that is too fast to allow stabilization on any particular psychiatric medication.

When we have a patient in whom we have found an infection and we want to treat them, we have to be mindful that they are not going to have time to get stabilized on any particular drug because as we treat them their symptoms may change too quickly. We need to be able to adapt more rapidly and hopefully get people through the process much faster so they don't need psychiatric medication in the first place.

SHARON

I used the CES after an unexpected death in the family. I had fallen into a depression and the anxiety had returned. I was on an anti-depressant, but needed a "boost." Dr. Stephen Xenakis, a psychiatrist, prescribed the CES and I found it helpful. I would lie in bed while Jeff was getting ready for work and I would run it for two cycles. By the time I kissed him goodbye, I felt less anxious about my day, and more willing (and able) to start my day.

At night, I used it on the lower settings to quiet my brain and thought patterns. It was another piece of my nightly routine to help me settle down and prepare for sleep (which did not come easily for me for many years).

For me, the CES was an introductory tool to meditation. Eventually, it got me to where I could quiet my mind enough to try meditation tapes.

SECTION SEVEN

PHYSICAL THERAPIES FOR HEALING

"All you have to do is look straight and see the road, and when you see it, don't sit looking at it - walk."

– AYN RAND

PHYSICAL
THERAPIES

There are numerous types of physical therapies that can aid in the healing process from chronic illness. Each of these is helpful in a unique way; it's important for each patient to find what works best for them.

Also, the phase of treatment can alter the outcome, so

if you tried something once before and it didn't

work, it might work for you now or later in

the course of the illness or treatment process.

The following section was written by Kathy Pesavento, MSPT, DPT, CMTPT

Issues Common Among Lyme Patients

A common thread for all patients is a level of fatigue and poor stamina that is new and unfamiliar to them. Usually patients will limit their physical activities and rest more due to this fatigue. Muscles can quickly become deconditioned and weakened, which can make any physical exertion that much more difficult.

A vicious cycle then ensues—the less you move, the weaker and tighter the muscles get and, conversely, the weaker and tighter your muscles are, the less you want to move. Bad postural habits begin, along with altered gait and movement patterns. Patients may begin to favor a part of the body that hurts and unconsciously change the way they move, for example, when climbing the stairs, or changing the amount of weight they put through each leg when walking. An imbalance of strength and tension in the muscles from one side to the other and/or from front to back can thus result.

The human body is balanced and symmetrical. This balance or symmetrical strength and flexibility on all sides of a joint is what keeps that joint stable. So, although Lyme Disease can affect the joints themselves, joint pain can arise from such imbalances in the muscles surrounding the joint.

Fascia

Not only are muscles affected by Lyme Disease and its co-infections, but connective tissue, called fascia, often becomes tight and restricted. Fascia is best described as a thin, flexible, and fibrous tissue that underlies our skin and encases organs, muscles, blood vessels, nerves, and other soft tissue structures in our bodies. Most of us have seen fascia—it is that thin layer of whitish, almost transparent tissue you see when cleaning a raw chicken breast. The fascia in our bodies allows organs, muscles, skin and other body structures to move and slide freely over one another, preventing friction from occurring.

Fascia also forms a three dimensional network in our body connecting virtually all internal structures together, so fascial restrictions in one part of the body can affect other parts of the body. With Lyme Disease, fascia often becomes hardened and tight, not allowing the normal excursion and movement of the tissues, organs, muscles, and joints and, in turn, causing tension and restrictions in the muscles and other tissues. There are several reasons why this happens.

Inflammation is one likely cause. Swelling causes increased pressure on surrounding soft tissue, which restricts its mobility resulting in discomfort or pain. Pain, in turn, causes the body to get inflamed in the area and a pain-swelling cycle starts. Chronic tension in both the muscles and fascia causes the tissues to become tighter and also limits the blood circulation to and from the muscles, which keeps the muscles from receiving proper nutrients and oxygen, as well as from eliminating waste products formed during normal metabolic processes. Once the muscles get tight, they in turn cause the fascia to get tighter. The muscles affect the fascia as much as the fascia affects the muscles. This is why the term "myofascial" ("myo-" meaning muscle) is used to describe tension and restrictions in both the fascia and muscle collectively.

Trigger Points

Chronic myofascial restrictions, which are very common in Lyme Disease, can lead to myofascial trigger points, or "knots," within a muscle. These trigger points, which are typically painful on palpation, feel like small nodules (often pea-sized) in the muscles and are best described as small, concentrated areas of muscle spasm, where the muscle tightens and does not release.

Several trigger points in a given muscle can shorten the muscle, making it weaker and less flexible and, in turn, cause decreases in strength and limitations in joint mobility. Trigger points can also cause referred pain or symptoms to other body parts. Other referred symptoms include numbness and tingling that can mimic disc herniation or nerve-like symptoms into the arms and legs. Trigger points can also refer pain to organs and conversely organ dysfunction can cause trigger points in muscles. And,

sometimes trigger points can mimic organ dysfunction without there being a true organ dysfunction.

Air Hunger

A common finding in patients with Lyme Disease and co-infections is the inability to either take a full breath in or exhale fully, coined "air hunger." Patients affected by this "air hunger" become very anxious that they may have a serious pulmonary or cardiac condition. But, in fact, it may be trigger points and myofascial restrictions in the muscles surrounding the ribcage and the accessory breathing muscles, which help us more fully inflate our lungs. A physical therapist trained in myofascial trigger point release should be able to more precisely determine the source of the symptoms and can quickly and effectively help patients regain most, if not all, of their breathing capacity.

SHARON For me, my air hunger was relieved in just four session of trigger point release therapy. It was a welcome relief.

Physical therapy, in conjunction with the proper medical and pharmaceutical treatment, is a very effective way to help decrease pain, increase function and mobility, and increase energy in patients with Lyme Disease and its co-infections. Physical therapy treatment plans are customized to meet each individual's needs based on their particular signs and symptoms. However, with the frequent and often daily change in symptoms, aches and pains, the rehab needs of a Lyme Disease patient will change, too.

Treatment Approach

Physical therapists need to be flexible in their treatment approach and realize that each day of treatment may bring a new adventure with each Lyme patient—both physically and emotionally. The goals of decreasing pain and symptoms, improving mobility and function, and increasing energy do not change.

Types of Physical Therapy

When diagnosed early, the Lyme and possible co-infections have damaged the muscles, fascia, and joints less. The body responds better and more quickly to rehabilitation. But, the more chronic the case, the more longer-lasting changes in the muscles, fascia, and joints. Unfortunately, many Lyme patients are misdiagnosed, sometimes for many years, and the disease may have caused the muscles to become more fibrous and calcified. This is accompanied by a significant amount of myofascial tension and restrictions. Treating these muscles and fascia is large component of physical therapy for Lyme Disease. Luckily, there are many "tools" a physical therapist specially trained in manual therapy can use to treat these chronically ill patients.

Manual Therapy

Myofascial trigger point release is a primary part of the rehab process. It can be achieved manually with the therapist using her fingers or assistive tools to place pressure on the trigger points in effort to have them soften or release. It can be done passively by simply compressing the trigger point until it softens (called "ischemic pressure"), or the therapist can have the patient contract and relax the affected muscle while applying manual pressure to the trigger point until it releases.

Another even more effective technique of trigger point release is *dry needling*. Trigger point dry needling is an invasive procedure whereby a solid filament needle (or acupuncture needle) is inserted directly into a trigger point in order to release it. There are different schools of thought on dry needling, but the desired effect is a twitch (or sudden, involuntary contraction) in the muscle. The needle is withdrawn slightly (not pulled out of the skin) and redirected to fan around the area of the trigger point until all the twitching has subsided. It is the twitching that ultimately releases the trigger point. The needling can be uncomfortable and typically results in muscle soreness for approximately 24 hours and, less frequently, some minor bruising, but is by far the most effective way to release trigger points.

As compared to manual release, the needling is longer lasting or permanent, relieves pain more quickly, and can get to deeper muscle structures that are difficult or impossible to reach manually with the therapist's fingers.

Needling is not for everyone due to personal anxieties, a low threshold to pain, or other medical conditions. Your therapist will determine if you are a good candidate for this procedure and you ultimately have to give your consent before beginning needling. Not all states have passed legislation allowing physical therapists to perform dry needling within their scope of practice. So, dry needling is not available everywhere. As needling is an invasive procedure, it is advisable to seek a therapist with extensive training and experience.

Fascial (or myofascial) release specifically targets the tension and restrictions in the fascia, and is another key technique to use on patients. Fascial restrictions can be more superficial and restrict

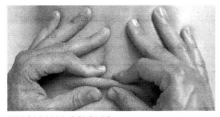
MYOFASCIAL RELEASE

skin mobility how well the skin can move over the underlying muscle and soft tissue. A physical therapist can quickly assess skin mobility to determine the extent and direction(s) of the restriction.

There are several manual techniques to release these restrictions, including *skin rolling,* where the therapist pulls the skin away from the body and rolls through or plows it along the restricted area. A small plunger or suction device can also be very helpful in pulling the skin away from the body to break through any adhesions or restrictions in the fascia. Cupping is also a common way to pull the skin away from the fascia. Such superficial treatment of the fascia can have deeper implications as some fascial restrictions may run deeper or farther into the body, causing pain or stiffness elsewhere.

Fascial restrictions involving the organs (or viscera) can be released with a technique known as **Visceral Manipulation**. It is a gentle and passive technique that helps to eliminate or lessen fascial restrictions around the organs to allow them to move freely in all directions as they do in normal functioning.

Strain Counterstrain is another commonly used technique to release tight, tender muscles. It is completely passive and is safe to use on most any patient. Best of all, it can be taught to a patient as part of a home program for them to do independently outside of therapy. It is a technique that requires positioning a patient to achieve the shortest position of a given (tender) muscle and maintaining that position for ninety seconds, allowing the muscle to "reset" itself and release. Again, the fact that it is passive and pain-free is very appealing when working with a patient with Lyme or its co-infections as often the inability to tolerate treatment can slow the rehab process down.

Therapeutic exercise

Exercise is an important part of rehab for chronically ill patients. This can range from stretching and flexibility exercises, to strengthening, postural, range-of-motion, and endurance exercises. Again, this is dependent on each individual's needs.

At a minimum, stretching and flexibility exercises need to be primary in a patient's home program due to the stiffness that accompanies Lyme. Also, after any type of trigger point release, stretching exercises are a must to get the best possible effect from the manual or needling release. These exercises will also help to prevent further trigger points from occurring in the same muscles. Strengthening exercises can help with muscle weakness.

Strengthening exercises must start off as gentle exercises since the muscles are deconditioned. It is important to address core (trunk and pelvic) muscles in a strengthening program as core strength not only is essential for appropriate extremity training, but also because it helps to alleviate back and abdominal weakness and pain, which are common in patients.

Functional exercises are basically normal daily routine activities (or components of them) that can be performed repetitively to increase strength and endurance in a way that the muscles will be used, such as climbing stairs, squatting to the floor to reach for objects, or even rolling over in bed. More aggressive aerobic exercises can help to increase overall stamina and individual muscle endurance.

Walking is a great exercise, either outdoors in the fresh air or on a treadmill for a more controlled environment, where compressive forces on all the weight bearing joints, such as the back, hips, knees, ankles, feet, can be lessened by slightly elevating the treadmill to a low degree of inclination (one degree works in most cases).

Biking is another good non-weight bearing modality for those who have joint pain while standing. An even better non-weight bearing exercise is swimming. Swimming is also a great aerobic exercise and is helpful in increasing cardiorespiratory endurance. If swimming laps is not possible or too aggressive, walking laps in the water is incredible as a strengthening, endurance, and functional exercise. Walk forward, backward and side-to-side. Starting in lower-level water (like thigh-height) and progressing to waist-height and eventually chest (or lower ribcage)-height water as tolerated is a good way to increase the level of difficulty.

Modalities

Other "tools" that physical therapists can use to treat Lyme patients, to name a few, are modalities, such as ultrasound, electrical stimulation, cold laser, moist heat, and cold packs to name a few.

Ultrasound uses sound like a sonogram but is set for therapeutic benefits, such as increasing circulation, decreasing inflammation, and heating the soft tissue. It is a great tool to use to loosen muscle and decrease pain.

Electrical stimulation is the application of low levels of electrical waveforms delivered via electrode pads placed on the symptomatic area. The sensation experienced by the patient can be like tingling or "pins and needles" and sometimes may make the underlying muscles contract and relax like a kneading massage type of feeling. Often times electrical stimulation is combined with simultaneous moist heat or cold packs in the physical therapy office to either aid in muscle relaxation (using heat) or relieve pain and swelling (using ice).

A TENS (Transcutaneous Electrical Nerve Stimulation) machine is a type of electrical stimulation device that is portable and a wonderful way for patients to get pain relief at home during flare-ups. They can either be rented or purchased, but have a physical therapist recommend a unit,

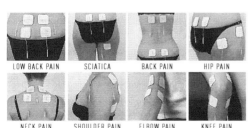

LOW BACK PAIN   SCIATICA   BACK PAIN   HIP PAIN
NECK PAIN   SHOULDER PAIN   ELBOW PAIN   KNEE PAIN

TENS ELECTRODE POSITIONING

set it, and instruct you on its use prior to you trying it independently at home as there are certain precautions and contraindications when applying electricity to the body.

Cold laser is another modality that helps to soften muscle tissue with the intent of releasing trigger points and muscle tension and also to decrease joint pain and inflammation by increasing circulation and promoting tissue healing. It is completely passive, pain-free, and non-invasive. When treating muscle tension and trigger points, it offers a wonderful alternative to those patients who either can't tolerate dry needling or manual trigger point release, are afraid of needles, are not candidates for dry needling possibly due to medical status or history, or are not working with a therapist who is trained in dry needling.

How to Find Help

Not all therapists are created equal. Finding a good physical therapist skilled in myofascial release and manual therapy is a critical step on the road to recovery. Historically, most physical therapy schools have not focused as much education on treating muscles and fascia as they have on treating the joint and surrounding tendons and ligaments. It is the continuing education courses, required in most states for therapists to maintain their physical therapy licenses, where therapists learn more specialized skills to better enhance their clinical abilities.

Some therapists may not necessarily advertise their skill set, but don't hesitate to ask a potential therapist about her training and manual skills background. Although there are advantages to seeing a therapist who is really good at one technique, there is no guarantee that that technique will work for a patient. A therapist with a more diverse skill set has more "tools" that may help. Getting a good referral from a medical provider, friend, or even an online referral service in your community is the best way to find a skilled therapist. Word-of-mouth referrals are usually based on personal experience, so those people can offer good insight on that particular therapist. A list of physical therapists is also available on the American Physical Therapy Association website—www.apta.org.

OTHER PHYSICAL THERAPIES

Acupuncture

When standard treatments like ice and heat, anti-inflammatory medications, physical therapy, and appropriate exercises can't ease the pain associated with chronic illness, acupuncture is an option with a good track record that's worth considering.

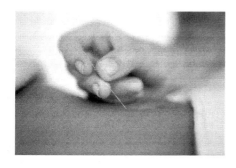

Over the years there has been substantial debate about whether acupuncture really works for chronic pain. Research from experts indicates that it does provide real relief. In 29 studies involving nearly 18,000 participants, some had acupuncture, some had "sham" acupuncture, and some didn't have acupuncture at all. Overall, acupuncture relieved pain by about 50%. The results were published *in Archives of Internal Medicine. ("Acupuncture for Chronic Pain", October 22, 2012; Andrew J. Vickers, DPhil; Angel M. Cronin, MS; Alexandra C. Maschino, BS; George Lewith, MD; Hugh MacPherson, PhD; Nadine E. Foster, DPhil; Karen J. Sherman, PhD; Claudia M. Witt, MD; Klaus Linde, MD).*

Acupuncturists insert hair-thin needles into the skin at specific points around the body. It is virtually painless when done by an experienced practitioner. Inserting the needles is thought to correct imbalances in the flow of energy in the body, called qi (pronounced "chee"). These pathways _**do**_ correspond to anatomical nerve, lymphatic, and vascular pathways.

I used three different acupuncturists in seven years of treatment. I encourage patients to find an acupuncturist they like and they find effective. It is also good to try it during various phases of treatment.

The following was written by Dan Parrish, LAc, NCCAOM

It is quite possible Sharon's success with me later in her treatment was because her general toxicity had greatly lessened by the time she came to me. When the toxic load is high, the symptoms are obviously greater. The patient is often overwhelmed by the toxicity and the effects they have on the digestive and/or neurological system. In this stage the acupuncture and herbs are often an adjunct therapy to antibiotic therapy.

Acupuncture alone, at this stage, can be like trying to put out a forest fire with a glass of water, as the symptoms are severe and often require western medicinal treatment. Often the patient has not been prescribed antibiotics for more then a few weeks, or they need an alternative to prevent being on antibiotics for a long time. Chinese herbs can help with the toxic overload and its ill effects.

There are herbs with anti-microbial effects, that support the immune system, that support lymph drainage and detoxification to help remove toxins and die-off from the system, as well herbs that can breakdown the bio-film.

Chinese herbs also address individual specific patterns of meridian disharmony. Each patient has a unique pattern of excesses, deficiencies, strengths and weaknesses that can be determined by tongue and pulse diagnoses. These patterns of disharmony must be corrected; clearing the toxins is not enough to deal with the complex imbalances chronic illness causes to a person's body mind and spirit. Even all non-Lyme patients have unique imbalances and these previous imbalances and constitutional strengths and weaknesses can determine how the disease effects them and to what degree.

Practitioners of Chinese medicine are trained to recognize and correct these imbalances, but it is far more difficult to find an acupuncturist/ herbalist who has experience with Lyme and co-infections. Lyme related illnesses make up about 25% of my practice since I live and work close to the Appalachian trail in Virginia. I have learned quite a bit, not only about what herbs can attack what bacteria, but also how the acupuncture needs of a *Babesia* patient differs from a person suffering from *Bartonella*.

Like Chinese herbs, the acupuncture addresses the unique patterns of disharmony that all patients have but are often greatly magnified with Lyme related illnesses. Correcting these imbalances helps to increase circulation, reduce inflammation, calm emotional upset, regulate the immune system and assist in their bodies' ability to heal itself again.

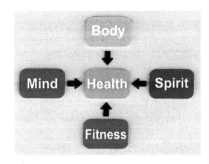

When the patient is in the throes of the disease I often use acupuncture to lessen the symptoms, which also helps lessen the patients' reliance on pharmaceuticals. I have had significant success limiting the pain, improving sleep, digestive functions, and neurological issues. As the person improves, the focus shifts from clearing toxicity and controlling symptoms to treating the long-term patterns of disharmony. The more balance we can achieve with the body-mind-spirit the better the person can avoid future flares and return to a healing path.

The following section was written by Daniel P. Hockstra D.C., AFMCP

Chiropractic care

"Shoulders of Steel" is the first thing that ran through my mind when I was honored to be asked to include a section in *Lyme Savvy*.

Bacteria, such as spirochetes are what I tend to call "bugs" when speaking with patients with Lyme Disease and the associated co-infections present with pain and stiffness throughout the joints and body. Pain can be referred by muscles, tendons, ligaments, fascia and bone.

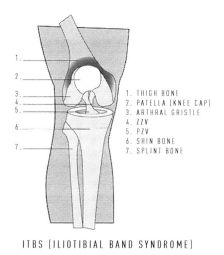

1. THIGH BONE
2. PATELLA (KNEE CAP)
3. ARTHRAL GRISTLE
4. ZZV
5. PZV
6. SHIN BONE
7. SPLINT BONE

ITBS (ILIOTIBIAL BAND SYNDROME)

As a chiropractor, I see most patients reporting discomfort in the greater thoracic girdle; between the shoulder blades, the neck and shoulders themselves. The second most common site is the ITB or iliotibial bands that connect the lateral side of the hip to knee in the legs contributing to potential full lower extremity dysfunction when compromised. The tissue will be extremely congested but not inflamed like most acute muscles or discogenic (referring from disc or nerve) injuries.

Picture the skin of fried chicken; the shiny layers between the muscle bellies and other connection points is called fascia. Fascia is a natural padding system between and around muscles that allows the body to make complex dynamic movements like swinging a tennis racket or golf club or getting out of bed in the morning. Fascia buffers the friction that muscles can create when moving across each other and connects muscles from the head to the toes in amazing spiraling patterns.

In the Lyme patient, this fascia feels as though it has turned into

Velcro layers encompassing the muscle. In cases where Lyme has been undiagnosed for years the adhesions become so great that sclerotogenous pain patterns commonly present. This is pain referring not from the muscle as seen by trigger points or nerve as seen in dermatomes or radicular pain patterns, but the tendon, ligament, fascia, vertebrae and joint complexes. Once restrictions are formed in spinal joints the nerve flow can also be inhibited. Spinal and extremity joint restrictions can cause neurological deficiencies, as well as pain and dysfunction in organ systems. Gentle chiropractic adjustments mobilize joints that are locked or restricted, increasing the range of motion of the joint and reducing muscular and lymphatic congestion and overall reducing pain in the area.

Adhesions

Adhesions form when the lymphatic system cannot drain fluid out of tissue in the body. This is seen after an injury like a sprained ankle, when the joint swells with nutrient rich blood and fluid that will eventually be used to heal the injured tissues and trigger pain receptors to fire and stop the individual from further injuring the structures. The fluid that does not get reabsorbed causes muscles and fascia to bind together with microscopic chunks of scar tissue or adhesions.

These adhesions will be disorganized, almost like taking parallel lines and laying crosshatches over them. As the adhesions lay down, the tissue will get further congested, often physiologically shortening the muscle tissue and tightening the structures. The saying "if you don't use it you will lose it" does ring true here. A reduced range of motion will be seen in all the affected tissues and the joints they move. The chronic spiral really begins at this point, as inflammation is the true cause of adhesions in the body and "bugs" naturally create low-level inflammation.

The acute Lyme case commonly presents with hot or warm joints that tend to travel, chasing the pain. The chronic Lyme patient slowly gets stiffer and stiffer with malaria-like cycles of pain and dysfunction. Patients may present with small flair ups on a daily cycle where the evenings will be the most aggravated, while others may have weekly, monthly or even yearly flair ups often mixed with Herx reactions.

The natural cytokine reaction the body uses to kill off bad cellular invaders can become too prolific with the kill off of bad cells. The body's trash removal system can not get the dead cells and gunk out of the system fast enough and results in increased myofascial pain flair ups along with other flu like symptoms. Any old area of weakness in the body will be more vulnerable to flair ups during these times and it can be different for each patient.

Patients with chronic adhesions are unusually characteristic because the tissue will get extremely tight and rigid but not be inflamed on palpation. Other muscle dysfunctions with nerve compromise like MS or ALS will feel totally different and tend to be boggy on touch between the shoulder blades and other areas near the spine because the health of the nerve is being compromised in a different way.

In Lyme Disease, it is almost as though the "bugs" have changed the short arch contractions of the muscles actually affecting the fiber recruitment and rate coding of the muscle fibers. Shoulder muscle tension in many patients could almost be reported in tensile strength as seen in engineering or evaluating steel itself. "Bugs" can create overall muscle pains most commonly in fibromyalgia-based sites, where two or more muscles cross in different directions or vectors with high concentrations of lymphatics in the same area. As one muscle gets tight over another it will cause friction that will grow scar tissue or adhesions in the area and further inhibit lymphatic drainage.

Chiropractic Techniques

Chiropractic adjustments can be an effective way to co-manage Lyme Disease and co-infections by mobilizing a restricted or locked joint. Adjustments are used to get a stretch inside the joint or vertebral complex stimulating alpha motor neurons that relax deep joint based tension.

There are over 300 different chiropractic techniques. All adjustments can stimulate the inside of the vertebral complex in ways that can make the nervous system work better and without interference. Providers can have an assortment of chiropractic tables from flat benches to machines that move left and right for the torso and upper extremity, flexion extension of the low back and spinal distraction. When full spinal adjustments are performed in combination with myofascial and fascia work, the most optimal results are expected.

Check out your local state association for chiropractors in your area. American Chiropractic Association http://www.acatoday.org

Diversified Technique

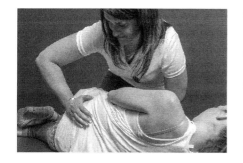

This is the most commonly used chiropractic technique. The patient lies in a comfortable position on a well-padded table while the practitioner puts a gentle impulse or motion into a joint to generate movement and thus adjusts a specific segment. The patient may lie on their side and the chiropractor brings one leg bent and forward and puts pressure on the sacrum and crosses the patients arms giving counter pressure to rotate the spine and adjust areas from the pelvis, sacrum, coccyx or lumbar spine. A "crack" or audible may be heard, releasing a pocket of nitrogen gas from the joint but is not needed to adjust and move a restricted joint. This will also bring blood flow into the locked joint to promote a reduction of stress and tension in the joint and surrounding tissues.

If the patient is not relaxed enough, the potential benefit of the adjustment will not be achieved. It is important the patient feels comfortable with the chiropractor and/or any manual therapist in order for optimal goals to be achieved because these are all physical touch based therapies.

Thompson Drop Table/ Pelvic Blocking and Craniosacral Therapy

Thompson Drop technique is an adjusting technique using a specific table that raises portions of the table from ½ to 1 inch then drop lightly by applying a specific directional force. This can be a very effective way to get an adjustment in spinal joints with the kinetic energy generated by the table giving way. The patient tends to feel less of a thrust because of the drop piece of the table. The adjusting table can usually rotate laterally, separating the upper and lower body at the hips or midline as well as flexion and distraction of the lower back. Pelvic blocks and boards can be added to help the provider be more specific and or incorporate Cranio-sacral techniques.

Craniosacral Therapy

Craniosacral therapy uses the provider's hands and focuses on the head and the base of the pelvis or sacrum as points of contact to enter into the nervous system and help unwind neural and dural tension on the spinal chord. This can be a very powerful combination to mobilize deep fascial and dural adhesions. http://www.upledger.com

Adjusting Instruments

The Arthrostem, Impulse and Impulse IQ are examples of vibration hand held adjusting tools used in Lyme patients to get the deeper adhesions in the facet joints that are located lateral to the vertebral end plates called myofibroblasts. Specific healing vibration frequencies are held over time to restricted joints to manually break up these nasty adhesions that traditional chiropractic adjustments cannot reach. These adjusting tools have been described as feeling like a mini jack hammer. Tension, pressure and vibration frequencies are controlled by the practitioner with different interchangeable attachment heads for separate areas of the spine and body. These tools are used with different adjusting styles.

Activator Methods

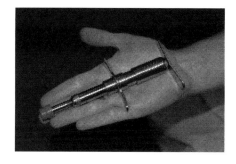

This is the most commonly recognized gentle or light adjustment technique. The practitioner will have the patient start face down on a padded table. Specific protocols are used to check landmarks like leg length differences where one heel is shorter than the other while the patient is not weight bearing. The provider will use a small pain-free adjusting tool that "clicks" to adjust the full spine in a very objective methodical manner checking for body alignment inequalities. The table often lowers you from a standing position to face down. This is another very gentle pain-free technique and is a good starting point to stimulate neurological changes in severe Lyme patients. (http://www.activator.com)

Active Release Technique or A.R.T.

A.R.T. is a patented myofascial technique of protocols to release adhesions and nerve entrapments where adhesions grow up into peripheral nerves that cause radicular like referring pain patterns in the body. The muscle or tissue is shortened and then actively lengthened while the provider places a translational force at the correct depth and in the direction of the tissue that needs to be reorganized. Imagine having a rubber band with a knot. When the rubber band is stretched the knot gets smaller but still exists. A.R.T. goes after that small knot (scar tissue) to break up adhesions within the Lyme tissue.

A.R.T. is a very effective hands-on therapy for patients particularly when performed with chiropractic adjustments to mobilize congested joints. A.R.T. does not have to be painful and is often described as a really good deep stretch/massage. Bruising of the skin can happen, although uncommon. In most Lyme cases after 1-2 days post treatment the patient will feel the most relief. www.activerelease.com

SHARON

I went to a chiropractor for decades before my *Bartonella* diagnosis. For most of those years, his Diversified method was immensely successful. In the later years, I think the inflammation got so bad it finally became ineffective. I couldn't get "cracked" anymore.

Once the inflammation was reduced, I went back to regular adjustments, grateful for that "cracking" sound again. It always brings immediate relief.

There are several different types of chiropractic care offered. Make sure you find what works for you.

Massage Therapy

Most people are familiar with deep tissue massage or Swedish massage therapies. But most chronically ill patients cannot handle an intense massage. The fascia and muscles are usually too constricted to be able to tolerate it. Below are descriptions of alternative massage therapies I found helpful and healing. Some worked better than others and again, it depended on where I was in treatment. I have since been able to go back to deep tissue massages, but it took a lot of fascia release and consistent massages to be able to get to this point.

Lymphatic Drainage Massage

Lymphatic Drainage massage is a gentle style of massage that focuses on assisting the lymphatic system into moving the lymph more effectively and efficiently. Lymphatic Drainage massage helps stimulate and support the immune functions of the body. It is highly beneficial to the patient for the support of the immune system and it is gentle enough not to increase any pain the body.

Thai Massage

Thai massage aligns the energies of the body using gentle pressure on specific points. Thai massage also includes compressions and stretches.

You don't just lie there–the therapist moves and stretches you into a sequence of postures. Thai massage is more energizing than other forms of massage. It is also improves flexibility and range of motion. Thai Massage combines techniques including Trigger Point Treatments, Myofascial Techniques, Neuro Muscular therapy, and Manual Therapy.

The combination of energetic and physical aspects makes Thai Massage unique. Traditional Thai massage is a deep, full-body treatment, starting at the feet and progressing up to the head. Using a sequence of gentle, flowing exercise movements, the recipient's body is moved, loosened and stretched of the joints and the muscles. This type of massage influences the energetic side as well, restoring the flow of energy throughout the body with applied acupressure on the sen energy lines of the body, aimed at harmonizing and energizing.

Believed to be over 2000 years old, traditional Thai massage is a healing art and a form of body therapy developed by people who used massage not only as a therapeutic method of healing to treat illnesses, but to maintain health and well-being. It is the combination of yoga stretching, calmness of meditation, with acupressure, exercise movement and reflexology that makes it a healing art. It is worked on a floor with the client dressed in comfortable loose clothing. Thai method uses mainly point pressure and muscle stretching. And it is not only the hands that are used to free tension stored in the recipient's body, but the feet and elbows are used as well.

There are various levels, so if you have pain, make sure your therapist knows you need a very gentle Thai massage.

Reflexology

Reflexology involves applying pressure to certain reflex points on the feet and hands that correspond to organs and systems in the body. Reflexology has many known benefits of relaxation,

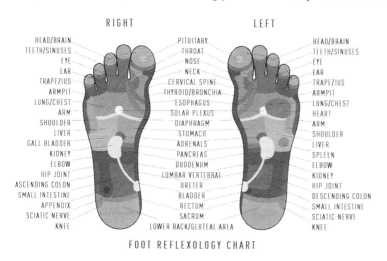

FOOT REFLEXOLOGY CHART

improving circulations, and relieving pain. Reflexology tends to relax the entire body through its ability to calm down the sympathetic nervous system (fight or flight response) and to assist the parasympathetic nervous system (resting, maintenance and nourishment of the body) to function more efficiently.

The feet and hands have specific reflex points corresponding to every organ, gland, cell and body systems. Stimulating a reflex nerve ending on the feet and hands sends a message to the corresponding organ, gland, or body system resulting in increased blood, nerve, and lymph circulation - and leading to improved functioning, enhanced cell nourishment and more efficient elimination of metabolic waste products. Working with all the reflex nerve points on the feet and hands gives your whole body a system a "tune-up."

Reiki

Reiki is an ancient method of hands on healing that was re-discovered in the 1800's by a Japanese Buddhist Monk. "Reiki" means Universal Energy. It is transferred to the person desiring

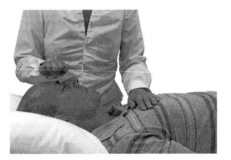

healing by a trained practitioner whose energy field has been aligned with the Reiki vibration through a series of attunements. These attunements are passed down to the practitioner by a Reiki Master.

Reiki works on all levels of the human body: the physical, mental, emotional and spiritual. It helps relieve pain and acute symptoms – strengthens and harmonizes the immune system. Reiki is believed to always act wherever the person receiving it needs it the most. Reiki is felt as having an innate intelligence that knows where to go in the body.

It has been known to alleviate some symptoms of Lyme Disease ostensibly by balancing the energies in the body—strengthening the immune system and life force energy-reducing stress-releasing patterns and blocks to suppressed emotions and promotes natural self-healing.

Reiki enhances personal awareness and spiritual growth, necessary for any healing.

Yoga

If you have never tried Yoga, I encourage you to read this section with an open mind. Yoga is not simply a bunch of women sitting around looking beautiful. It's a workout. The beauty of yoga is:

- the intensity is decided by the participant,
- the practice of yoga involves so much more than "poses,"
- every single pose can be modified for the participant's restrictions, thus making it something anyone can do,
- effective breathing is taught and refined throughout classes,
- relaxation is an essential element to yoga (yoga nidra)

There are several types of yoga. The key is to finding not only the right type of yoga, but also the right teacher. Don't give up too easily on this.

After three years of treatment, I finally had the strength to start "working out" again. I chose yoga as my first step. I approached a local studio owner, explained my story and she recommended a few classes based on their style and the teacher.

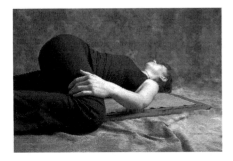

Restorative Yoga is directed towards students who are injured, stressed or ill, who need a very gentle practice and who are looking to rogain the quality of life that they used to have. It involves the use of props (sometimes lots of props) to allow the body to feel totally supported, to allow the body to relax and release; long holds of these gentle postures, postures often selected to address specific challenges; and deep mental and visceral relaxation. Restorative Yoga takes an unhealthy body and brings it (hopefully) back to normal. It is important to tell each teacher beforehand what your physical limitations are.

In a Restorative Class the size of the class is much smaller than most yoga classes, perhaps four to twelve students. This allows the teacher to get to know the health and injury status of each student and thus tailor the poses and options for each individual. The whole class is usually quieter and more relaxed than other styles of yoga classes.

Yin Yoga is <u>not</u> intended to be Restorative Yoga. Yin Yoga's purpose is to take a normal healthy body and bring it up to its optimum. It encompasses long held, static stresses of the deep connective tissues allowing them to be remodeled. It offers significant opportunity for fascia release. It usually includes props and it does include long holds and mindfully reducing stress but it is not intended to heal broken bodies in the way that Restorative Yoga does.

In an arguably average sized Yin Yoga class, say fifteen to thirty students, the teacher is going to focus on the average condition of the majority of students: catering to the extremes is rarely a successful strategy for teaching yoga - if offering poses that only the most advanced student can do, there is a higher risk of boring or possibly injuring everyone else; however, if the poses are safe enough and easy enough for everyone to be able to do, many students can become bored. If the teacher is experienced she can layer the class into several levels to offer something for 90% of the class, but no teacher in one class can offer something for every possible health condition.

Again, I was gifted with a teacher who helped me modify uncomfortable poses to something more healing for my body. I was able to take Yin Yoga for a few months when I could do nothing else. Even though I wasn't a "normal" or "healthy" person, Yin Yoga was key to stretching and preparing my muscles for healing.

NON-TRADITIONAL TREATMENT MODALITIES

SHARON

For various reasons patients may seek remedies in a variety of alternative treatments. Some may not have good experiences with traditional treatments. Some patients choose non-traditional modalities for political or religious beliefs. Others elect these methods because of health benefits they have previously reaped from those modalities. Many patients use non-traditional protocols to complement the traditional treatments. They find it makes a good combination or "one two punch." Some of the non-traditional practices are excellent at reducing symptoms or side effects.

And some patients choose some of these modalities out of sheer desperation. Nothing else has worked, so why not try them? Here, we highlight some of the most popular non-traditional methods used by Lyme patients.

DR. MOZAYENI

Hyperbaric Oxygen Therapy (HBOT)

There are a few important things about hyperbaric oxygen. Air is 21% oxygen and the rest is mostly nitrogen. A hyperbaric chamber will increase the delivery of oxygen and nitrogen to cells. At 100% oxygen under 2.36 atmospheres (2.36 times normal pressure at sea level) the concentration of oxygen is about 11x higher thus

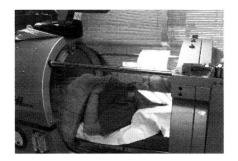

the delivery of oxygen to tissues is much higher than the oxygen provided by air at the same pressure and because much of that oxygen can now also be delivered in the blood and not just carried by the red cells, the tissue delivery of oxygen becomes even more greatly enhanced than even the math would suggest.

When we administer hyperbaric oxygen we have to consider if there are neurological symptoms. If so, one has to start with lower pressures, typically 1.5 atmospheres. This is because as the partial pressure of oxygen increases, blood vessels constrict. Your body will reduce blood flow to an area If the level of oxygen in the blood goes up; because you are delivering more oxygen, blood vessels constrict to compensate and regulate the amount of oxygen getting in. As you increase the partial pressure of oxygen there is almost a proportionate constriction of the arteries to reduce blood flow to an area. This can also transiently relieve migraines and increase blood pressure.

This constriction of blood vessels, though temporary, can worsen the neurological symptoms. This is a very important point. In a patient who has Lyme Disease, the tendency has been to try to use very high pressures of oxygen ostensibly to kill *Borrelia (Lyme)* microbes. This was all based on a study of about 15 people done by Fife (Fife Protocol). Most all of those patients were worse during treatment. The assumption has been that the *Borrelia* are actually killed by very high pressures of oxygen. We all know that Lyme testing has never been good enough to really know that you have actually eliminated all of the *Borrelia.* We cannot actually verify whether or not the high pressures of oxygen that are usually used are actually effective at killing the *Borrelia* because the *Borrelia* tests have not been good enough.

Furthermore when one has neurological problems, it is a medical mistake to be using pressures that are too high. Always one should start at lower pressures and gradually work up and probably never exceed two atmospheres of 100% oxygen.

Currently, we have absolutely no idea how sensitive *Borrelia, Bartonella, Protozoa,* or any co-infection may be to high partial pressures (concentrations) of oxygen. The lab tests available until recently have not been able to sensitively detect these bacteria. So we have not had good before-and-after studies to see if the high-pressure oxygen actually works for various co-infections, and these studies will likely not be funded in the foreseeable future.

Many of the centers providing hyperbaric oxygen therapy for Lyme Disease often treat with pressures that are too high and can cause neurological complications and worsening cognition. Potentially, in an inflamed blood vessel that is more prone to spasm, a little extra constriction caused by higher concentrations (partial pressures) of oxygen could even cause a stroke. One has to be very careful and really re-think why and how we use hyperbaric oxygen in Lyme Disease. It is only from a good understanding of the physiology that one can then start to draw conclusions about when and how it can help.

Even at the slightest increase in oxygen pressure, one can induce the production of many new hormones and growth factors. And, you reduce inflammation and hyper-coagulation. Many of these mechanisms have been studied. There is documentation of least 3,000+ genes or biochemical reactions that are enhanced with hyperbaric oxygen.

With hyperbaric oxygen therapy the benefits are broad as many healing processes are activated by oxygen at high concentrations achieved with pressurization. New science shows we can reliably use hyperbaric oxygen to increase stems cells and induce repair pathways and help rehabilitate a patient. This includes patients who have micro-vascular injury to various tissues including their brain. Parts of the brain that sustain transient loss of blood flow from small-vessel disease will develop 'stunned' or 'idling' dysfunctional neurons. These neurons are not dead; they are not functioning well and could be resuscitated potentially with oxygen. Similar mechanisms apply with benefits in traumatic brain injury, so whether it's from physical trauma or vascular trauma there are nerves that function poorly and these may be reactivated and restored to function with safe low-pressure (low dose) hyperbaric oxygen.

We need more research to fully document and validate these benefits and to optimize the timing of how we use HBOT. However, the general clinical experience is that in most HBOT facilities that treat patients with chronic illness, it is generally favorable but can have some side effects in the short term. I think side effects can be mitigated considerably if the facility recognizes it is more effective to use it as a repair and rehabilitation modality than an antimicrobial germ-killing modality.

Bartonella and *Protozoa* like *Babesia*, manifest many symptoms through their effect on the vascular system. The infection is primarily in the vascular system. The associated symptoms may be attributed to what the microbes are doing to the vascular system. The biofilms associated with these germs line the blood vessels, float around, and impair the circulation. Because these germs really like to be in the vascular system where they like to live on and within red blood cells, it is unlikely they are very sensitive to oxygen because they live in the vascular system where oxygen levels are the highest. Therefore, the idea that you would use hyperbaric oxygen to treat germs that like to live inside your vascular system doesn't seem plausible – unless future studies or extensive clinical experience show, using newly advanced microbe tests, that high oxygen pressures achieved by HBOT can kill these germs.

There is also data regarding *Borrelia* that upon exposure to oxidative stress, the *Borrelia* immediately become dormant cyst forms. There was an *invitro* study done by an NIH group in Colorado where they exposed *Borrelia* to hydrogen peroxide (Murgia and Cinco 2004). Upon exposure to a small dose of hydrogen peroxide, the *Borrelia* turned to cyst forms. Therefore, hyperbaric oxygen may cause the *Borrelia* to go dormant as cyst forms. There may be transient temporary improvement by making the *Borrelia* go dormant then we are not actually killing the *Borrelia*. At very high pressure concentrations, we might be, but no one has been able to look at that with advanced lab tests. The testing has not been good enough to be able to even design those experiments for *Borrelia*. Again, this research, too, is very unlikely to ever be funded.

The newer improved culture methods for *Bartonella* and the new highly sensitive *Borrelia* tests may now allow us to do such a study. I think as the molecular detection methods for the *Protozoa* improve we may be able to see if the *Protozoa* are sensitive to very high concentrations of oxygen.

Going forward, we need research to determine how effective an HBOT protocol would be in wiping out some of these bacteria – a protocol that starts low and gradually builds up to higher pressures. In the meanwhile, I think it should be used principally as a modality for repair and rehabilitation and not as expect it to be a modality for these chronic infections.

Hyperbaric oxygen is a simple therapy. You apply a simple life-giving molecule but at higher doses and pressures than normal. You need to understand the physiology of what is happening because patients could be feeling a lot worse needlessly in receiving hyperbaric oxygen therapy. Lyme patients have come to think that unless they are feeling worse, they are not going to get better. A lot of what they are feeling in the hyperbaric chamber may not be a "Herxheimer" reaction at all. It may be that the high pressures of oxygen cause blood vessels to constrict and reduce blood flow and thus, worsen neurological symptoms.

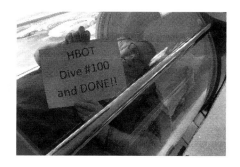

Because of that, hyperbaric oxygen therapy should perhaps be used towards the end of antimicrobial treatment. Oxygen may even support the growth of some of these germs because we know these germs like oxygen. They live in the vascular system. I believe it best to use HBOT later in the course of treatment to help people recover from the entire disease process. HBOT may help reduce inflammation after antibiotics are started.

The entire treatment process needs to be individualized with the caution that if there are significant neurological symptoms, pressures should be kept low and then maybe later, increased as tolerated.

The clinical science of all this is in its infancy and for now it remains an off-label protocol. Given that the FDA now regulates hyperbaric oxygen as a drug, it is highly unlikely that there will ever be sufficient funding for a study to obtain a new FDA 'label' for hyperbaric oxygen therapy.

Essential Oils

Essential oils can have anti-inflammatory, analgesic, and potential anti-microbial properties. The best oils with these properties are Oregano, Thyme, Clove, Cinnamon, Eucalyptus, and Tea Tree. Essential oils should always be diluted with a carrier-oil as they can irritate sensitive skin. Apply over entire body after a daily shower or bath.

Some essential oils can be quite powerful and if used improperly can cause more distress than aid.

The Calming oils are gentle, sensitive, and can be used with little to no adverse reaction. These oils include: lavender, blue chamomile, sandalwood, patchouli, and lemon balm.

The Energizing oils have awakening properties. Use these oils in the morning or when feeling sluggish. Sweet orange, lemongrass, frankincense, peppermint, and rosemary are some of the Energizing oils.

Stimulating oils should be used sparingly on the body. Many of them have antibacterial and antiviral properties. The Stimulating oils include marjoram, juniper, basil, thyme, and cinnamon.

I found the essential oils to be helpful in relieving symptoms of my condition, but I would not consider them as a sole protocol for curing Lyme Disease or any co-infections. Remember, essential oils should never be internally ingested.

DR. MOZAYENI

Rife Machines

Rife machines were originally developed in the 1930s by Royal Raymond Rife. The general notion is that an electromagnetic current can be used to interfere with a disease process and in particular to kill microbes. The thinking around rife machines has evolved to the point where the hypothetical premise is that germs have a specific electrical frequency, and that by interfering with that frequency, one could kill the microbes, suppress the germs and allow the body to heal.

I have never been able to see or to find or to evaluate any data that demonstrates that the application of electromagnetic frequencies actually can kill these various microbes. There may be some examples that could be used to counter this statement but the problem really isn't so much the scientific premise as it is the validation and calibration of any instrument that is put out there with that intention.

There are other types of electromagnetic devices that claim to be able to measure and capture the electromagnetic frequencies of not just germs but also the energy of particular supplements. They claim to be able to assess your electrical field and then determine based on that what sort of supplement you should take. Whenever I have asked for simple calibration data showing me how the instrument is tuned to be able to do what they perform as it is described, there has been no data to be found or provided to me.

Because we do know that atoms, molecules, proteins, and cells have electromagnetic fields and electromagnetic properties it is theoretically possible that at some point someone may develop a very advanced device that can do some of these things. So far, I have not seen any data or any convincing information even that these devices can really work. The claims are entire "word of mouth," and I am sure some people have had a positive experience using these methods.

The FDA classifies many of these devices as consumer devices, meaning that they think these devices don't do anything so they don't need to evaluate and regulate them. This further implies that they these machines are unlikely to be doing anything helpful. Some patients may disagree and everyone is entitle to their opinion.

The first question I ask whenever I am asked about these instruments is, assuming they could work at all, "How do we know they are well calibrated?" No matter how advanced your scientific instruments – even the most advanced scientific instruments known to mankind – have to be calibrated.

If all of these devices that are so advanced and so effective must be calibrated, how is it that something that could selectively knock out microbes in your body or adjust and manipulate disease process in your body would not have to be calibrated?

Most of the time consumers and even clinicians are not in any position to be able to adequately evaluate the validity of any of the statements provided by practitioners or manufacturers of electro diagnostics. I have had on occasion been in a position where I have known that the claim is wrong simply because what they claimed to be able to do has not yet been possible scientifically, to calibrate.

For example, some of these devices claim to be able to detect the presence of *Bartonella* electro-diagnostically. Since I know there was no method available to detect *Bartonella* in a patient conclusively (based on the research that I was personally involved with), I knew that the instrument could not possibly do so. I simply knew there was no way to calibrate the instrument to do what was claimed.

Electromagnetics are used diagnostically and therapeutically in medicine but I don't think there is sufficient science to use these principles to diagnose or treat microbes. You will see devices that are intended to treat or claim to treat a condition, as well as some that claim to be able to diagnose a condition. I also know physician colleagues who have micro current devices. The effects that a patient might get from a micro current device could be helpful in theory, but it is not yet reliable or generally applicable because there is no scientific framework around it.

If you apply some sort of electromagnetic field to your body it changes the body's electromagnetic fields. Even sitting next to an electrical outlet on which there is electromagnetic pollution from solid-state electronics can have some effect on you. Therefore it might fall into the category of things that change your physiology and your biochemistry and therefore alters a disease process somehow. But it's not a scientific process. It's not one that has been established to have a calibration or validation of its effect.

With diagnostics it is always important to ask yourself "What is the best measure of the truth that I have and how closely does this diagnostic tool come close to our best assessment or measure of the truth?"

I was involved in developing a diagnostic device. One of the people we met with for some advice was a former director of the FDA. The first question he asked was 'What is your measure of truth, in this instance, and how does your diagnostic device calibrate or measure up against your best estimate of the truth?'

Many users of these electro diagnostics will also complement the diagnostic process with natural and herbal therapeutics. Although these remedies may be helpful, the inaccuracy of the data is offset by the fact that the herbal remedies alone may have helped or the herbal remedies in connection with other modalities might have helped too. Studies comparing these various therapies are needed.

At best, the biggest downside is that these treatment options distract you. If harmless and they make you feel better to go through the process then there may be some placebo value there. But recognize that it's also a distraction from where you could **more productively** spend your time, energy, and resources.

Magnets

The issue with magnets is interesting because there is a new form of FDA-approved electromagnetic therapy, which is called the Pulsed Electromagnetic Frequency device (PEMF). We think it induces a form of intracellular 'exercise' so to speak. It has been referred to as 'magnetically induced cellular exercise (MICE)'. It has been shown to help reduce some pain syndromes and it may be helpful in some way with patients who are chronically ill. But as far as I know its only uses have been to treat pain syndromes. The therapy is based on pulsed electromagnetic frequency.

We call it electromagnetic because electrical fields induce magnetic fields and magnetic fields induce electrical fields. An electromagnetic wave, which is a radio wave or an electrical wave, is propagated through a wire or space by one field alternatingly inducing the other. You have a magnetic vector in the field and you have an electrical vector. As these fields are alternating, oscillating fields, they are characterized by their frequency (cycles per second, Hz).

A magnet produces a static magnetic field. A magnet by itself does not oscillate and produces only a fixed magnetic field. If you move something through it like a wire you would induce electrical movement in it. A magnet placed on a part of the body has been anecdotally used by consumers to help with healing and pain locally on a particular part of the body. I have not seen any medically convincing case.

Personally, with bad knee injuries and sprains, I never felt it made any difference although I tried it with an open mind. It's important to understand that a magnet itself is a static field, a magnetic field; that it is not an electromagnetic field. And relative to the Earth's native magnetic field, an individual magnet may not be significant. The Earth has an oscillating electromagnetic field. A book, *Earthing*, has been written on potential benefits.

Alkaline Water

In general, practitioners treating chronically ill patients tend to recommend what we call an alkaline diet.

One of the complementary products marketed to many patients is alkaline water. The premise being that if you drink enough alkaline water, you will create more alkalinity in your system. Creating more alkalinity helps your blood flowing more smoothly. If your pH is low you are more likely to coagulate. Your blood is more viscous, it's thicker, it's more prone to clotting; your circulation is going to worsen.

Alkaline is good and alkaline water certainly isn't bad. The main question is if **alkaline water is effective <u>compared to</u> some other way for you to alkalinize yourself**.

I have worked in research laboratories where we used ultra pure water, which we called 10 mega ohm water; the mega ohm is the amount of resistance that the water provides to electrical current. Most people don't realize that water is not a good conductor of electricity if it is completely pure. What *does* allow electricity to move through water are dissolved minerals and salts including calcium, sodium, chloride, etc.

If you are doing a science experiment where you are applying an electrical current to water, you add salt (saline). You put salt in the water to make it a better conductor of electricity. But in a research laboratory when you want ultra pure water you remove all of the minerals from it until it is an extremely poor conductor of electricity. Most salts dissolved in water have a buffering capacity.

The buffering capacity of water depends on what's dissolved. In the human body, the major buffer is phosphate. Secondarily, it may be carbonate, other salts, and all the proteins and amino acids that are in the system.

The normal pH of the body is about 7.4. The body goes to great trouble and has many redundant systems to carefully adjust and maintain that pH balance. If your pH dropped quickly from 7.4 to 7.1, you would be very sick. It would take a major illness, like kidney failure, poisoning, or trouble breathing, not putting out your carbon dioxide, that might cause your pH to go down. Even very small pH changes are a very big deal for biochemical reactions.

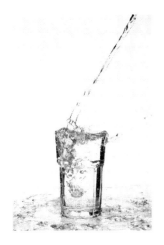

When considering water, you have to consider not only its pH but its buffering capacity. You could have acidic water that has no buffering capacity and it would do absolutely nothing to your pH. In other words, if you had alkaline water that had a low mineral content and thus, lower buffering capacity, it would do absolutely nothing to your body pH.

If you alkalinize your water and it has no buffering capacity, then you have wasted your time because it is not going to affect your pH at all.

Interestingly, and paradoxically,

organic acids like citric acid (lemon juice) and acetic acid (vinegar) do more to make you more alkaline than alkaline water.

You are not likely to get much buffering capacity out of alkaline water unless it is high in mineral content. Some mineral waters, especially the sparkling ones, have a much higher dissolved mineral content. Unfortunately most mineral waters tend to have a significant amount of sodium.

While alkaline water may be helpful, if it has buffering capacity, there are better ways to alkalize the body. And, if the water was highly alkaline, it would increase stomach pH and that would reduce the efficiency of protein digestion.

SECTION EIGHT

DIETARY RECOMMENDATIONS

"Let food be thy medicine and medicine be thy food."

– HIPPOCRATES

The Simplest Changes to Make

If the details in this chapter are too overwhelming to incorporate, consider these as the simplest measures for nutritional support in your healing:

1. FODMAP diet – Educate yourself on the FODMAP diet and incorporate into your dietary habits

2. Reduce arsenic levels by removing or cutting back on chicken and brown rice

3. Avoid farmed salmon if possible as most have PCBs.

4. Eliminate mercury – Remove tuna and swordfish from your diet

5. Cut out histamine producing foods such as nightshades and fermented foods

6. Uncover hidden food allergies – Specifically eggs, dairy, soy and wheat (gluten)

7. Eat more greens and vegetables.

8. Avoid sugars and simple starches.

Testing for Food Allergens

Food sensitivities have the potential to cause all of the symptoms that you might otherwise attribute to Lyme Disease. This is because food sensitivities stimulate systemic inflammation; a host-response. Clinicians and patients need to look at food sensitivities and find ways to manage them. If this is ignored or overlooked, you may be attempting to treat Lyme Disease when, in fact, you have a food sensitivity.

Feeling lethargic after eating is a typical indication of food sensitivity response. If you eat the same food each day you won't know it is from that particular food because you feel continuously fatigued. In fact, even if you do not eat the offending food one day, you may not notice any difference in how you feel because it can take weeks to recover.

Food sensitivities can be significant — the smoking gun for many patients. The problem is that insurance only pays for the IgE antibody tests for foods that cause anaphylactic shock, such as peanut allergies, so you should request and receive IgG- or IgA-based tests. IgG tests are usually done through specialty labs and are not reimbursed by insurance. And remember, in some cases, more advanced testing is needed — such as measuring the cellular immune response through specialized labs — if the antibody testing is unrevealing.

It is far easier to do the blood test and see if antibodies are present. While the antibodies don't prove an allergy with certainty, it is a way to begin your search. It really helps narrow things down. You should eliminate anything that is positive on the report, including anything that flags as even slightly positive. Once you have found and eliminated the foods causing reactions, you need to avoid them completely for several months before slowly adding them back in to your diet, one at a time.

The good news is if you avoid the offending foods for long enough, your immune system may become desensitized. Once that happens, some people are able to occasionally have those foods again with little or no reaction. This prolonged avoidance can be highly transformational and helpful in recovery from chronic illness.

Food sensitivities are particularly common in patients with chronic conditions. They may have been pre-existing or maybe the inflammation caused a so-called leaky gut, which broke the mucosal barriers. It's possible those antigens would have gotten in one way or the other whether the gut was leaky or not. The immune system may be hyper-sensitized so it is cross-reacting with food antigens. Food sensitivities cannot be overemphasized for their importance in treating chronic illness and their effects on a person's health.

The Big Four
There are three or four food categories that some doctors will often recommend eliminating from a patient's diet even without testing simply because the likelihood of a food sensitivity is far greater with these four items. They include: wheat, dairy, soy, and eggs.

OTHER IMPORTANT FACTORS

Enzymes

Enzymes help break down proteins and help reduce viscosity and improve blood circulation.

There are enzyme-based supplements: Bromelain, Papain, Lumbrokinase, and Serrapeptase. In my experience, enzymes are very helpful in minimizing symptoms and making treatment more tolerable. Enzyme-based therapies that help improve circulation are important not only to relieve symptoms but also to improve treatment success.

Fresh fruits and vegetables contain enzymes. Cooking destroys the enzymes' functions, so be sure to eat fresh, raw, uncooked fruits and vegetables.

Pickling is a way to preserve enzymes and produce probiotics. The pickling fluid's low pH acetic acid helps preserve enzymes. A lot of pickling is enabled by certain probiotic organisms, which create the sourness in the fermentation process. Apple cider vinegar as a pickling agent, combined with enzymes and probiotics, helps to alkalinize your body and reduce inflammation.

Alkalinization

An alkaline diet is low in sugar, as sugar tends to be acidifying. Organic acids like Vitamin C (ascorbic acid) or even vinegar (acetic acid), are alkalinizing inside the body even though they are chemical acids. Ascorbate Vitamin C is also antioxidant and an alkalinizer biologically. The best way to alkalinize is through diet; you will attain a higher alkaline buffering capacity and alkalization through the metabolism of organic acids. A tablespoon of apple cider vinegar, or having a salad with this amount of apple cider vinegar as a dressing, will assist in alkalinizing the body.

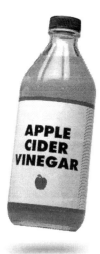

Apple cider vinegar, like any organic acid such as citric acid (lemon juice) or Vitamin C ascorbic acid, biochemically becomes an alkalinizer, not an acidifier, after it is metabolized. It is not straightforward chemistry; it is bio-chemistry. If the vinegar contains sugar, it will be acidifying when the body metabolizes it. The take-away is that balsamic vinegar is slightly acidifying; apple cider vinegar is alkalinizing.

You can alkalinize your system not just by carefully choosing foods and avoiding sweets but also by eating vegetables, sources of organic acids.

Vitamin C Alkalinization

VITAMIN C

Even more effectively, you can alkalinize with high-dose Vitamin C.

One can test weekly to see how much Vitamin C is needed. This is known as bowel tolerance Vitamin C. Once weekly, take a few grams of Vitamin C every 30 minutes to an hour. You will eventually have loose bowel movements because your bowel will stop absorbing the vitamin C. This stage will indicate to you that you have reached your threshold. For the rest of the week take 75 percent of that total.

Let's say it took 20 grams to give you a loose stool. For the rest of the week you will take 75 percent of that, 15 grams, and spread it out over the course of the day. You might do 3 or 4 grams four times a day. What does this achieve?

- It boosts your immunity.
- It reduces your coagulation.
- It reduces inflammation.
- It is an antioxidant that is water-soluble.

When this is joined with the antioxidants that are fat-soluble, you move the free radicals and oxidative by-products from the lipid environment (cell membrane) into the water environment, which is then excreted by the kidneys.

Vitamin D

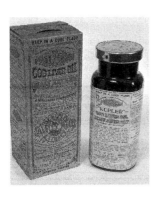

Vitamin D is a sterol made from cholesterol and a hormone produced by your body with ultraviolet light.

Be aware that this process requires direct sunlight-to-skin contact; vitamin production does not occur if you are behind glass and only when the sun is high in the sky. **In the winter, from September to March, nowhere north of Atlanta, Georgia, are you able to produce Vitamin D from direct sunlight.** In some parts of the world, Vitamin D is from the diet because people ingest high quantities of seafood or cod liver oil. Norwegians, for example, have among the most stable seasonal levels of Vitamin D worldwide, despite a varying annual northern sunlight schedule due to their position near the Arctic Circle.

Vitamin D is an immune hormone and an Interferon booster among other things. Achieving good Vitamin D levels will provide you with significant immunity against numerous viral infections. We monitor Vitamin D levels carefully and have found the incidence of flu in patients of mine who take Vitamin D regularly is significantly lower than those who do not. Exceptionally low levels may cause muscle aches and bone pain that can mimic fibromyalgia.

There are two forms of Vitamin D, vitamin D2 (ergocalcifero) and vitamin D3 (cholecalciferol). If you produce a lot of the Calcitriol form

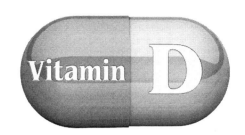

(1,25 OH- Vit D), the activated form, it may be a clue that you still have inflammation. This is because the enzyme making the active form of Vitamin D is found in some immune cells. Thus, Calcitriol can be an inflammation marker in some cases.

If you have inflammation you have to be careful not to take too much Vitamin D all at once but to build up slowly. Dr. Holick at Boston University, the leading Vitamin D expert, recommends adults and children alike receive between 4,000 and 6,000 units per day. I have seen people's needs vary from 2,000 up to 10,000 units a day; those with high stress levels and obesity generally needing more. Toxicity is generally not a concern as you would need 6-12 months of 10,000 units to come close to being toxic. However, if you have inflammation, taking too much Vitamin D too quickly can produce too much of the 1,25-OHD3 which could cause additional symptoms.

Ideally, we also want to avoid using synthetic prescription Vitamin D2, which is dosed at 50,000 units once weekly because it is synthetic and may interfere to some degree with normal Vitamin D3 metabolism. Its efficiency in conversion to D3 is only about 30%. When you start taking Vitamin D, start with half of the low-end dose, maybe 2,000 units a day, and let it build up slowly. As you start feeling better consider increasing the dose and monitor the

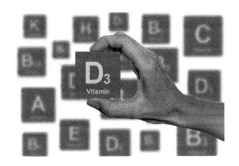

blood levels; aim for mid-normal levels of Vitamin D3.

Stress activates cortisol production and cortisol accelerates the breakdown of Vitamin D. Many chronically ill patients end up spending a lot of time indoors, which prevents them from receiving the sun exposure, they need. Combining these factors, they now have stress and limited sunlight resulting in accelerated Vitamin D breakdown and no new Vitamin D production. As a result of the illness they may also become Vitamin D deficient, leading to more new symptoms, including osteo-malacia, signified by bone and joint pain. This domino effect causes further confusion in the evaluation and management of Lyme Disease.

Protein

Protein is necessary for repair. I don't think it's possible for the human body to survive on a pure vegan diet if you are recovering from a chronic illness. Consuming animal protein is necessary for certain sterols or amino acids, which are not prevalent in plants. There is an array of quality protein sources. Egg whites are known as the gold standard protein while some people like fish, though you have to be careful not to eat large predator fish because they contain toxic levels of mercury.

DR. MOZAYENI

Other Nutrients Needed

There are certain key nutrients that you will not obtain from plants:

B12 - If your diet is low in red meat then you must take B12. This applies to most everyone because people are not eating red meat as often.

Biotin - Biotin is normally made by the healthy bacteria in the gut. It is vital to carboxylase enzymes and is important in the integrity of skin, hair, and nails, as well as important in the immune system's fight against yeast and fungal infections. If one is on antibiotics, as long as the biotin levels are kept up, you are at reduced risk for yeast infections. It is my recommendation that anyone taking antibiotics should be supplementing once daily with biotin, a relatively inexpensive and easy solution. Also be aware that egg whites will significantly bind and reduce biotin.

Juicing

Juice is basically a green smoothie with the fiber removed. Fresh green juices are an opportunity to load up on nutrients at a high density. Juicing with fresh crisp vegetables is a great way to ingest enzymes, Vitamin C, and sulfur; it also conveys to heavy alkalization. Juice is a powerful nutrient-dense elixir that is healing, energizing, and significantly health-promoting. Juicing is excellent for those who have trouble processing fiber and for those who have severe gastro-intestinal issues.

You consume a higher mass of produce when you make juice. This makes juice more expensive by volume — another point to consider — but you acquire more nutrition in this condensed form. Juicing is mostly for the "green" vegetables; not many fruits.

A juicer is less expensive than a good blender for green smoothies, but the amount of vegetables you use for your juicing is at least five times the amount you would use in a green smoothie.

Be careful, in that juicing can create a high-caloric food and unless you leave the fiber in, you can lose much of the nutritional value. It is best NOT to drink prepared juices from the store as these are too calorie-dense, depleted of fiber, and may contain unhealthy byproducts.

Green Smoothies

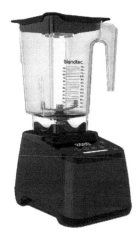

Green smoothies are made in a high power blender such as a Vitamix, Kitchen Ninja, or Blendtec with little to no waste of the actual fruits and vegetables that you use. If you are looking to get more nutrition in your diet but you don't want to spend a lot of money on the produce, then consider green smoothies versus juicing. Green smoothies also have the advantage over juicing with cleanup being easier and faster.

Fiber goes a long way to form bulk in your colon which helps bind toxins including heavy metals, cytokines, and a lot of inflammatory mediators — reducing your general health risks, overall inflammation, and risks of colon cancer. It also adds volume to a green smoothie that fills you up using only a fraction of the produce you would use if you removed the fiber and drank it as juice.

Many find green smoothies to be more tolerable by adding unlimited amounts of berries, or lesser amounts of certain fruits due to high sugar content, to disguise the taste. Unlike juicing, when making green smoothies, you are able to add protein powders and chia or flax seed. Because of the myriad options and ways to make green smoothies more flavorful, children are more likely to drink them rather than green juices.

If you would like to lose weight, the fiber bulk in smoothies make them very filling as a super healthy, low-calorie meal replacement.

THREE WAYS STRATEGIC EATING CAN IMPROVE YOUR HEALTH

The following section was written by Robin Shirley, CHHC

Nutrition can play a far greater role in your recovery from chronic Lyme disease than most of us currently believe. I know this because I myself have used nutrition strategically to eliminate approximately 50 percent of my symptoms without using any other treatments. I have now tested this protocol on dozens of clients who have also reported that when they change their diet, using my guidelines below, many of their symptoms that they once thought could only be resolved with medical intervention and strong antibiotic therapies, simply fade away.

The three main reasons for this are:

1. Conventional food contains impurities, chemicals and toxins that weaken our immunity, impair our hormone and energy synthesis and block detoxification pathways, causing headaches, rashes, fatigue, impaired sleep, inflammation and neurological and muscular dystrophy.

2. Nutrient-dense foods contain the compounds needed to strengthen our immune system to fight infection.

3. Nutrient-dense foods contain antibiotic compounds that can fight infection directly.

I: THE FOODS AND FOOD IMPURITIES THAT WEAKEN YOUR BODY & IMMUNITY

There are some foods that either weaken the body directly, in the case of common food allergens, refined sugars, and trans fats, or they are contaminated with toxins that weaken the body, including heavy metals, preservatives, and pesticides. When you eat these foods you are putting an unnecessary burden on your immune system, which distracts it from focusing on fighting the Lyme infection and co-infections.

Food Allergens: Food allergens are a surprisingly significant cause of symptoms in Lyme disease patients. Food allergens are foods that cause an immune system reaction, leading to symptoms like headaches, fatigue, depression, irritability, disturbed sleep, rashes, joint inflammation, nervous system inflammation, dandruff, itchy skin, and more. The reason these foods are causing this reaction is that many of us have damaged digestive tracts, and some of the protein molecules in these foods are being allowed to pass, partially undigested, into the bloodstream. The immune

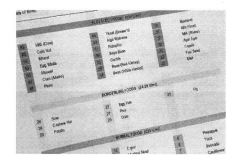

system considers intact proteins to be foreign invaders, and will attempt to destroy and remove them from your bloodstream.

Common food allergens that Lyme patients should definitely avoid include gluten, dairy, soy, corn, and eggs. I go into more detail about the causes of a damaged digestive tract and why these foods are a problem, more than any others, in the GMO section.
Food allergens are causing significant symptoms in almost 95 percent of the Lyme patients that I work with.

If you want a clear picture of which symptoms are actually being caused by the disease and not by your food, you must eliminate food allergens.

Doing so can eliminate or significantly reduce a high percentage of your symptoms, at which point you'll be able to see which symptoms remain and can be attributed to disease. I see many of my patients become almost 50 percent better when they eliminate the five common food allergens including corn, gluten, soy, dairy and eggs.

Once you eliminate food allergens, you may find that your symptoms are not as severe as you had thought, and your treatment protocols may reveal more positive results than before. Most patients are also able to think more clearly, be more productive and enjoy their lives more.

Genetically Modified Foods and Pesticides

Genetically Modified Organisms (GMO) food crops are ones that have been modified to withstand larger than average amounts of pesticides. If you look at the common allergens listed previously, you'll see that most of them are genetically modified, including soy, corn and dairy. Wheat (gluten), which is highly hybridized, is also heavily sprayed with the same pesticide (glyphosate) that is used on genetically modified crops.

There is a theory that GMO's are a contributing factor to the allergy epidemic because the pesticide (glyphosate) that is sprayed on most of them not only kills pests on the plant, but is sterilizing our gut, destroying our protective layer of gut flora and mucous, and allowing undigested food particles to get into our bloodstream. There, these particles are recognized as foreign invaders by our immune system, which launches and autoimmune-like inflammatory reaction.

Refined Sugar

Refined sugar is sucrose, fructose or glucose, refined from a plant source, bleached and stripped of its antioxidants and minerals. The resulting sweetener is usually white, light brown or light yellow, and free from fragrance. When you consume it, it gives you a ton of sugar, but no minerals, vitamins or antioxidants. So, you are stimulating your body to use energy through the sugar high you are giving yourself, but you aren't backing up that energy usage with nutrients that supply your body with the capability of producing that energy. So you are going into "energy and nutrient deficit." That's when you use energy that you don't have.

Another reason to avoid refined sugar is that it can feed pathogens when consumed in excessive amounts. Refined sugars include white cane sugar, white beet sugar, corn syrups, agave syrup and processed honey. Refined sugars are found in foods such as pastries, baked goods, bottled beverages, gums, candies, and some dried fruits.

Trans Fats

These are fat molecules that have been chemically restructured so that they have a longer shelf life or lend a specific texture to a food. They are "rancid" and cannot lend the same nutritional benefit as fresh oils and fats. They act as free radicals in the body and do damage to your arteries and organs. Trans fats elicit an inflammatory response from the immune system, distracting it further from fighting the Lyme infection. Trans fats gave fat a bad name and should not be confused with unprocessed fats like tallow, lard, olive oil, butter, palm oil, and coconut oil, which provide essential cellular building blocks.

Plastics

Plastics contain chemicals that have been proven to disrupt our body's production of estrogen, progesterone, and testosterone. Because hormone balance is so essential to immune function, detoxification, and energy production, Lyme patients must be especially careful to eliminate hormone-disrupting plastics. These plastics get into our body through our skincare products, food storage containers, which leach plastics into our food, water bottles, and more. It is essential for us to stop storing our food in plastic containers, but if you must, at least do not use them to store hot foods or liquids. Use glass or glazed-ceramic containers instead. You should also switch to a reusable glass water bottle and organic skincare products.

Heavy Metals

Heavy metals are extremely damaging to human tissue. They cause free radical damage, which your immune system has to spend time and energy repairing. They also block hormone uptake receptors and detoxification pathways. Heavy metals like lead, mercury, cadmium and aluminum can appear in city tap water, bottled water, food storage containers, supplements, pesticides, medications and cosmetics.

Mold toxins

When ingested, mold toxins can suppress the immune system and cause unpleasant symptoms including skin rash, headaches, impaired brain function, liver stress, and digestive upset. For the first reason alone, Lyme patients should strictly avoid foods contaminated with mold toxins. Mold toxins can be found in coffee, tea, peanuts, and some dried nuts grown in humid climates (especially cashews). You can still enjoy coffee and tea, just make sure to research and purchase brands that take care to reduce the mold toxins in their products.

2: EAT "SUPER FOODS" CONTAINING NUTRIENTS THAT SUPPORT YOUR IMMUNE FUNCTION

Body Processes Need Nutrients

Every single biological process carried out by your body is dependent on particular molecules including enzymes, proteins, and other nutrient compounds. These processes include blood filtration, hormone synthesis, muscle repair, white blood cell production, liver detoxification, feces elimination, energy synthesis, breathing, circulation, etc. The molecules that feed these processes are provided by nutrients that your body derives from the food that you eat.

We have to pose question, "Why do some people overcome the Lyme bacteria while others do not?" Certainly there are factors at play that we do not understand. But, could part of it be because your body is not being fed the nutrients that it needs in order to carry out normal biological processes to keep the body healthy? If you are providing your body, through the food that you eat, with the nutrients needed to carry out those biological processes efficiently, and without interruption, then your body should be able to fight the majority of infection on its own.

Adopting a diet that provides the nutrients that you need in order to fight infection on your own may sound too easy to some. Which is why nutrition has probably been overlooked as a serious step in fighting Lyme disease. And for those that have adopted certain dietary changes, they are probably not doing it correctly or intensely enough, or else we would have a lot fewer people suffering. These dietary changes are nothing to joke about!

The diet that I am proposing, the diet that actually provides the nutrients that your body needs to fight infection on its own, is not so easy at all. You've already seen how many foods you must avoid. This is not a "healthy diet" that you read about in Women's Health magazine. It is a very strategic diet and may seem exotic to some.

A body that is dealing with a chronic infection is a sick body and is nutrient-deficient. So, a "healthy diet" wouldn't even work in this case. You have to make your diet work "double time" for you because you are nutrient deficient and currently fighting a serious infection.

Necessary Nutrients to Fight Chronic Infection and Inflammation

We need to think about eating foods that are extremely nutrient dense. And we need to eat them on a daily basis. With every bite of food that we eat, we need to build our nutrient reserves for our body to use for important biological processes and for times of extra stress. You can't get that kind of nutrient-density from normal healthy foods. The calorie and fiber count in some common foods are too high for the small amount if nutrients they deliver. You wouldn't be able to eat enough of it to get the nutrient density required by your body.

Here are some particular nutrients that we need to start incorporating into our diets in higher amounts. And below I will outline particular foods that deliver these nutrients in generous amounts and realistic serving sizes.

Nutrients We Need In Generous Quantities:

Omega 3 Fatty Acids

These particular fats are beneficial for improving brain function including memory and for normalizing triglyceride and cholesterol levels. Good sources of Omega 3 fatty acids include hemp seeds, chia seeds, grass-fed beef, fish, krill oil, and blue-green algae.

Saturated Fat

This kind of fat has gotten a bad reputation in the media and common collective as a cause of heart disease. The studies that were conducted on the causes of heart disease found that saturated fat was a primary component of arterial plaque. Unfortunately, the studies stopped there. They never asked the question, "Why is the saturated fat there?"

Saturated fat is an essential building block for new cells. When your body is repairing blood vessel tissue, it needs saturated fats to build healthy new cells. Specific to Lyme disease, white blood cells depend on saturated fat for proper identification of foreign invaders including bacteria, viruses, and fungi.

Saturated fats are also used by the body to incorporate calcium into bone, to protect the liver from alcohol and drugs, and to carry out nerve signaling, among many other important tasks.

Good sources of saturated fat for Lyme patients include coconut oil and grass-fed beef.

Protein

Protein is used as a building block for every part of the body including muscle, skin, hair, and organs. Proteins are made of amino acids, which are precursors to immune response, cellular repair, hormones, and neurotransmitters. Neurotransmitters are responsible for brain function, such as emotional responses like happiness, and include serotonin, dopamine, and norepinephrine.

It is essential that Lyme patients consume enough protein to provide for all of these tasks. If a Lyme patient decides to eat a vegetarian or vegan diet, it is extremely important to watch the alternative protein intake, otherwise you will begin to see impaired brain and immune function and slow cellular regeneration.

Good sources of complete protein include grass-fed beef, pasture-raised poultry, wild caught fish, blue-green algae, hemp seeds, bee pollen, quinoa, and beans.

Carbohydrates

Carbohydrates are the preferred energy source of the body. If you aren't getting enough, your body will turn to protein or fat as an energy source, but it is an inefficient conversion and will result in toxic byproducts. It will also reduce the amount of fat and protein available to perform other essential functions that cannot be fulfilled by other nutrients. It is best to not deprive yourself of carbohydrates for too long, if at all, when dealing with chronic illness. Sometimes people will limit carbohydrates for training or for weight loss, but when you are chronically ill, I feel that it's best not to stress your body further.

Good sources of carbohydrates include winter squashes, quinoa, rice, vegetables, organic fruits (especially berries) and raw, locally harvested honey.

**Side note: Specific ratios of protein, to fat, to carbohydrates is a more advanced nutrition topic and is not necessary to track during initial phases of healing. In a chronic illness situation, first you must remove the foods that are damaging your body further and increase your nutrient intake across the board. Once you take care of those two steps and you are able to have the energy to take care of yourself, you can look towards the ratio of proteins to fats, to carbs to find an optimal balance for you as an individual.

Vitamins

Vitamins are organic compounds that are required by the body to carry out normal functions. Vitamins cannot be produced by the body in sufficient quantities and must be obtained through the diet.

Good sources of vitamins include fruits and vegetables, organ meats, kombucha, pollen, rice, quinoa, blue green algae.

Minerals

Minerals are naturally-occurring inorganic compounds that are required by the body for certain biological processes. They are not produced by the body and must be obtained through the diet. Good sources of minerals include organ meats, seaweed, chocolate, Himalayan salt or sea salt, blue-green algae, nuts and seeds, quinoa, rice, dark green leafy vegetables, and fruits.

Antioxidants

Antioxidants are molecular compounds that contain a specific combination of nutrients that repair tissue damage caused by oxidative stress, which is usually caused by radiation, carcinogens, oxygen exposure, and infection.

Good sources of antioxidants include richly colored and fragrant plant foods like herbs, seaweeds, algae, and fruits and vegetables.

Examples of "Superfoods" Containing High Levels of These Nutrients:

It is important to review a few specific examples of foods that provide exceptional levels of antioxidants, vitamins, and minerals per calorie. Many experts in the nutrition field call these foods "superfoods" because they are so extremely high in nutrients compared to the everyday foods you find on an average American dinner table.

These "superfoods" contain nutrients that are not found in adequate quantities in a standard American diet, and they are the nutrients that your body needs to fight infection, build hormones, repair tissue damage, and generate energy-producing hormones like cortisol and adrenaline. Here are a few examples of "superfoods":

Blue-Green Algae

This is a single-celled organism found in fresh water. It is a food staple in many countries, and has been for thousands of years. Blue-green algae is a complete protein, meaning it contains all of the essential amino acids (protein building blocks) that your body needs to get from food. Not only is it a good source of protein, but it also contains therapeutic phytonutrients including chlorophyll and astaxanthin. Chlorophyll assists the body with detoxification including blood purification as well as light detoxification of heavy metals. Astaxanthin is a powerful anti-cancer and anti-aging antioxidant. It has been shown to repair tissue damage caused by radiation.

Bee Products

This category of foods includes pollen, honey, and royal jelly. Pollen is the most nutrient-diverse and affordable of the three. It contains enzymes, which aid digestion, B-vitamins to support metabolism and energy production, antioxidants to repair tissue damage and fight cancer, and Vitamin C to repair tissue and support immunity. Pollen is also a complete protein and contains 40 percent protein by weight, more than any other protein source, including animal sources. Pollen is used as an anti-cancer and anti-aging tonic in Chinese medicine. It contains antimicrobial compounds and is effective against salmonella and some other strains of common bacteria.

Organ Meats

This is the part of the animal that is most dense in nutrients including iron, Vitamin A, and Vitamin D. Iron is needed to build red blood cells, which carry oxygen to our cells and feed our energy production. If you are at all anemic or low in energy, iron is an essential nutrient, and is best absorbed from animal meats. Organ meats are also a significant source of other trace minerals in addition to iron. Owing to our evolutionary past, humans are carnivores — best able to function when they are eating animal protein and fats. Vitamin A is a perfect example of why this is true, as it is a nutrient only found in animal food sources.

Plant-based foods are incorrectly labeled with "Vitamin A" content because they contain carotenoids, which can be converted into Vitamin A in the body, but are unfortunately only converted efficiently in about half of the human population due to a genetic mutation.

Even in humans without the mutation, carotenoids are converted at a low rate. So the amount on the food label is not what you are actually converting to Vitamin A in your body. Vitamin A is essential for skin health, eyesight, and immune function. Vitamin D is also an important nutrient for immune health and cancer prevention, and is only nutritionally found naturally in animal food sources, like liver and kidneys (the body can produce some Vitamin D from ultraviolet sunlight exposure).

These are just a few examples of my favorite "superfoods" for reversing nutrient deficiencies and building immunity and energy.

3: START EATING MORE FOODS WITH ANTIMICROBIAL PROPERTIES

The third way that food can support Lyme disease patients is through directly fighting pathogenic microbes with antimicrobial nutrients. This is where you can get even more strategic with your diet and use every meal as an opportunity to fight the Lyme infection and co-infections.

These are some examples of foods that contain nutrients that fight infection directly. They contain phytonutrients that actually act as antimicrobials and can bypass your body's ability or inability to fight infection.

Examples of Antimicrobial Foods:

High Vitamin C Fruits

This category includes Camu Camu berry, acai berry, rose hips, and mangosteen berry. These fruits contain exceptionally higher amounts of Vitamin C and polyphenols per calorie than other fruits, including oranges.

These nutrients boost immune function to support your body's own bacterial- and viral-fighting capabilities. They also contain antibiotic properties and fight infection directly. For example, Camu Camu berry is classified by the FDA as one of the most effective botanicals in combating the herpes virus.

Probiotic Foods

This category of food includes Kombucha, Kefir, and Sauerkraut. They are beneficial to Lyme patients because, unlike probiotic pills, they contain strong, thriving colonies of good bacteria, which rebuild gut flora and "crowd out" parasites and pathogens. Gut flora has most likely been destroyed in Lyme patients by antibiotics, pesticides on non-organic and GMO foods, food preservatives, a sterile diet, birth control, and other prescription medications.

Gut flora is essential because they produce B-vitamins, Vitamin K, and organic acids that rebalance the pH of our digestive tract. Gut flora also builds a protective biofilm and mucous layer on the surface of the digestive tract, which helps with digesting and filtering the food that gets absorbed into the bloodstream. Without this protective layer, we are absorbing partially-digested foods that trigger immune reactions in our blood, joints and nervous systems, leading to inflammation and food allergies.

Seaweed

This is a food that has been in the human diet of seaside cultures for thousands of years. It is high in absorbable forms of iodine, calcium, magnesium, and other trace minerals. Iodine is especially important for Lyme patients because it acts as an antimicrobial agent in the thyroid, where it is not only used to build the thyroid hormone, but it is used to sterilize the blood as your body pumps every drop of blood through the thyroid several times each day.

Culinary Herbs and Spices

These herbs include rosemary, basil, oregano, thyme, parsley, chive, garlic, cumin, clove, cinnamon, and more. The herbs contain phytochemicals and other nutrients that support the body with tissue repair, immunity, and hormone balance. The essential oils in these herbs also act directly on infection as antimicrobials.

Individual Health Challenges

You will need to take your individual health challenges into consideration as you work through changing your diet. Challenges including blood high blood pressure, diabetes, heart disease, blood clots, autoimmune disease, and cancer may require special dietary recommendations or considerations and with research and/ or consultation with your treating physician, you can use those together with my recommendations for Lyme disease and come up with a personalized dietary plan.

Don't feel as though you need to get everything worked out in a day. It may take years to come up with a comfortable eating plan, and it may take the assistance of many books, nutritionists, and doctors to get there.

If you take the time to learn a little bit each week, and make a few significant changes each month, you will be feeling the effects of your nutrition choices on your body in no time!

Eating Organic

SHARON

My first wake up call about the food I was putting into my body was when we got the first test results back, showing I had dangerously high arsenic levels.

"Do you eat a lot of poultry?" Dr. Mozayeni questioned.

"Yes, probably 3-4 times a week."

He referred me to a 2006 report by the Institute for Agriculture and Trade Policy entitled, "Playing Chicken – Avoiding Arsenic in Your Meat." I now eat only organic chicken and my test results show no arsenic in my body.

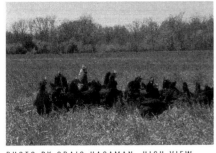

PHOTO BY CRAIG HAGAMAN, HIGH VIEW FARMS, BERRYVILLE, VA.

Buying organic chicken led to organic eggs, which led to organic vegetables. The process evolved from there. I used to think that "organic" was a way for the food industry to rip off the customer. I had no idea about genetically modified organisms (GMO foods). I didn't realize that so much of what I was putting into my body was filled with unhealthy ingredients.

When I was initially diagnosed, my husband started an organic garden in our back yard. I thought it was a sweet gesture, but I didn't comprehend the significance until we started eating what he had planted. We felt so much better after meals. The more research he did, the more grateful I became for his tireless efforts in providing organic vegetables for our family.

Jeff also started keeping bees on our property to help with pollinating our plants and to provide us with raw, unfiltered honey. I didn't realize what honey REALLY tasted like until I tasted the honey from our hives. WOW. If you usually only buy honey from the grocery store, please go to a local farmer's market or local organic store and buy *raw, unfiltered, local honey* (harvested within 500 miles of your home). But beware of the sugar and calories.

The dietary changes didn't come all at once. It was a step-by-step process. It had to be if it was going to be permanent.

I tried green smoothies as a last ditch effort to get my gut under control. And I found a way to make them that I enjoyed. I like the sweeter green smoothies. My husband likes the "nutrient dense" ones. And he likes to juice more than drink green smoothies. The important thing is that we keep trying these healthier alternatives and trying to find ways that will help us heal.

My greatest struggle remains with omitting refined sugar from my daily intake.

SECTION NINE

ATTAINING & MAINTAINING WELLNESS

"Being in recovery means having the willingness to stop running from emotional pain. It means that now we use this pain to learn, change, and grow into our fullest potential. Pain ceases to victimize us and begins to become our teacher."

– BARBARA S. COLE, *GIFTS OF SOBRIETY*

THREE PHASES OF HEALING: PHYSICAL, EMOTIONAL & MENTAL, AND SPIRITUAL

SHARON

Let me preface this section by saying that I do **_not_** believe there is a "dependency" or "addiction" issue among chronically ill patients. The following simply highlights one way I have utilized a program I was already in to deal with some of the issues that arose for me in my recovery from Lyme disease.

I am a recovering addict. I got sober in 1988 from a drug dependency to Valium, attending meetings of Alcoholics Anonymous. The process for staying sober was kept very simple: Don't drink, go to meetings, and work the 12 Steps of Recovery.

A simplified view of the process is that the healing takes place in three general phases: Physical, Mental/Emotional and Spiritual.

First, the physical part.

By taking the drugs and alcohol away, the body can start to mend itself and heal from the complications caused by ingesting harmful chemicals into the body on a regular basis. When the physical problems abate, progress can be made in other areas.

It is known that ingesting drugs and alcohol alter the brain's chemistry and thus functioning capabilities. After a few months or more of sobriety, the recovering alcoholic will notice they can "think better." The sense of a "brain fog" will begin to lift. This leads to the second phase of healing: mental and emotional healing.

For the alcoholic, this becomes a time to effectively "clean house," making amends for where they have injured others, accepting events that occurred in their own lives over which they had no control, and making an effort to live life on a positive, responsible, contributing level. This process can take months and even years.

Finally, when more of the "cobwebs" have cleared, the recovering alcoholic finds opportunities are often presented to him/her where a sense of spirituality will enter. They will see many "coincidences" occur that bring amazing gifts to their life for which they have no explanation. They find the more they trust in a Higher Power, the more able they are to live life with an attitude of gratitude.

For the chronically ill patient, these three phases of healing are titled the same, but are worked differently. These three aspects, the physical, mental/emotional, and spiritual, are worked concurrently.

Physical

Most of the physical treatment process is best, but not always, handled by the physician. This relates to the administration of medications and supplements, physical therapy, getting rest, getting blood tests. The medications have to get into the body to destroy the bacteria and to heal the body. Where the recovering alcoholic was removing things from the body to make it better (drugs and alcohol), the chronically ill patient needs to add things to the body to help the healing process.

This physical process is not as simple for the chronically ill patient as it is for a recovering alcoholic. The alcoholic has to stop doing things; stop drinking and taking drugs. The chronically ill patients have to **start** doing things. They have to start taking medications at regimented times. They have to rest often. They have to restrict their schedule. They have to reduce the amount of physical stress their body experiences. This requires an active participation and adherence to doctor's orders of what to do when and how to do it. This single task can sometimes become the most overwhelming for a cognitively impaired individual. It requires support from the patient's family and friends. It requires being able to go grocery shopping, preparing, and eating healthy foods. It requires procuring and dispensing medications on a timely basis without running out and going a few days without medication.

Mental & Emotional

The mental/emotional aspect of healing comes more easily as the body physically heals. It becomes easier to remember things. If the body is well nourished, the brain can function better. Therefore, it is easier to think clearly and make decisions based on better rationale.

Healing in this respect is NOT a matter of, if you think you are well, you will become well. It is not a "believe hard enough and you will get better" aspect. It's hard enough to heal, but when I hear from others if I "believe enough" that I will heal, it will happen. Sorry, it's not that simple. I can believe all I want, but if I still have bacteria and parasites in my body, it's not happening.

However, I do believe that attitude can be a game changer in the healing process. One of the first decisions I made after my diagnosis was that healing had to become my number one priority. It had to come before work, family, friends, everything. Every single task in my day became focused on this one goal.

For instance, taking my medications as prescribed. I set alarms on my phone to remind me to take my pills. And I took them, even when it meant getting up from a table of co-workers to get my purse and take them.

Healing meant scheduling rest time in my day. This was probably the most difficult task for me. I assigned "rest time" to being lazy. I had to re-label it "Healing Time." The body can only heal when it is at rest. So if I don't get enough rest, I will never heal.

I changed my daily schedule drastically. I had the luxury of owning my own business, so I was able to make my schedule more flexible. I went into work an hour later than usual, giving my body a chance to rest more each morning. I didn't necessarily sleep, but the simple state of lying horizontal (with my head level with my heart) allowed my body the restful state it needed.

I restricted all weekday evening activities. I did not go out after 5 pm. For me, my peripheral neuropathy caused me to fall easily. I tended to fall more easily when I was tired or rushing. And I was always tired by the afternoons. By restricting my activities to home in the evening, I had less likelihood of falling. Being home every night also afforded me the opportunity for less stress, not attending business functions, not having to interact with a lot of people. Staying at home each night was less of a brain drain.

On weekends, I allowed myself one activity for the entire weekend - that activity could be grocery shopping, attending our local farmers' market, coffee with friends, dinner out, or seeing a movie with my family. But I kept it to one activity a weekend.

I repeated to myself and others:

My number one job right now is to heal.

I allowed myself as many naps each weekend as my body craved. Sometimes it was two naps a day.

Because of the herxes, my body sometimes required me to stay in bed the entire weekend. I didn't cook, do laundry, clean house, anything. I sometimes had to simply lie in bed and do nothing. I couldn't read, write, knit, or needlepoint. I didn't want to talk on the phone, email, or get on Facebook or Twitter. I lay there feeling useless and lazy.

I remembered back to when I was pregnant and put on bed rest for the final ten weeks before delivery. I was agitated from the drugs and frustrated at being isolated and bored. I wasn't allowed to do anything. A friend then suggested that I develop a new perspective of the day.

"Every day you keep that baby inside you is a gift," she said. "Each day, you ARE working. You are creating kidneys, arms, eyes, fingernails. You are creating a baby inside of you." I could grasp that concept. Each day, when the frustration would start to build, I would read what parts of the body were developing and then I would focus my energy and attention to those parts. I participated in the process even if it was passively.

When I had to rest so much as part of healing from this chronic infection, I finally re-framed it as "Healing Time." My body WAS doing something. It was HEALING. And I needed to give it the **opportunities** it needed to heal. How I perceived this time was almost as important as giving myself the time. If I clouded my brain with worries, then how could my body be in a healing mode? There is a mind/body connection. Both must be in sync with one another for the healing energy to transform the body. It is all encompassing.

I remember one time when our family was trying to schedule a birthday celebration. This family member wanted to celebrate during the week. I told him I wouldn't be able to attend. It broke my 5 pm rule during the weekdays.

"Come on, you've got to be kidding me," he quipped. "You can't make an exception for one birthday dinner?" Pangs of guilt rose within me. And then I remembered the previous week when I was at the grocery store at 5:30 pm. I had stayed late at work to squeeze in a few extra things. At 5:30, with only half my list in my cart, I had to check out and come home. And I had great difficulty even doing that. Merely standing at the checkout line was formidable for me.

"No, I'm sorry. My number one job right now is Healing. Maybe we can make it next year when I am better," I replied.

Even though a birthday dinner is primarily sitting down and enjoying good food, it still required getting dressed up (at this point, I rarely applied make up in the morning or dressed in anything besides jeans and t-shirts because it took to much energy). It still required walking (with the possibility of falling). It still required social interaction (brain drain for me). It was in an atmosphere that often negatively affected my light and sound sensitivity, thus escalating my fatigue. I usually got home later than usual, and thus, get less sleep that night which then transferred into the next day's activities and energy levels (or lack thereof).

Thinking it Through

In AA, it's called "Thinking it Through." If you think a drink would be good, you don't just think about taking the drink. You think about what the one drink leads to, which is usually more drinks, then getting drunk, then saying something you regret, or doing something you shouldn't do, then waking up the next morning, feeling hung over, mouth dry, nausea, headache, then remembering what you did and what you said, the regret, the remorse, the anxiety and then trying to start the new day feeling so badly from the night before. It isn't pretty and usually the recovering alcoholic realizes they simply wanted some temporary relief from a very uncomfortable situation.

For chronically ill patients, they want to be "normal" and be able to attend events such as birthday dinners. But we are not normal and we have to "Think it Through" to see the total ramifications of our decisions and behaviors. We have to see how our actions will affect the "**new** normal."

Will This Help Me Heal?

Then we go back to, "Does this fit in with my number one priority of Healing?" If it doesn't, then we need to choose not to follow through on that decision. For me, some of my decision-making became greatly simplified.

"Do you want to go to the mall?" a friend would ask. My internal response became, "Is this task going to help me heal?" For me, going to the mall was, without question, extremely fatiguing. I didn't go to the mall for years. But I really wanted to spend time with this friend. Emotionally, I needed time with her. That would help my healing. I couldn't do the mall, but I could do coffee together for an hour. So that would be my compromise. I didn't have to lose the time with my friends, but I did need to readjust it.

Counseling

Sometimes, the emotional issues can become compounded with a chronic physical ailment. I needed a professional to help me through some of those issues.

A few months before I received my *Bartonella* diagnosis, I started EMDR therapy with a licensed therapist. I had been in talk therapy for years and found it helpful, but I still felt held back by certain incidents earlier in my life. A therapist recommended that maybe there was more to be done and that I might be suffering from a form of Post Traumatic Stress Disorder (PTSD).

Based on her recommendation, I saw this therapist who had outstanding results with using EMDR and SE (Somatic Experience) therapies. These therapies are discussed elsewhere in this book.

Spiritual

This is **not** a section about believing in God, or believing in anything "enough" to heal.

This is about opening yourself to the possibility of believing in a power greater than yourself and allowing that power to influence your life in positive ways. And I would even go so far as to suggest you might believe in multiple powers greater than yourself.

I am going to start someplace you might not expect me to: your physician.

By the time I found Dr. Mozayeni, I had been to at least 30 physicians in search of a diagnosis and treatment. I had seen some of the "best of the best," all came highly recommended by others who had great success in their own illnesses and recoveries. But none of them worked for me. I spent years trying to convince doctors something was really wrong with me to no avail.

When I finally found Dr. Mozayeni, putting my complete and whole trust in him was not a "natural instinct" for me. I had spent 30 years knowing something deeper was going on when many very well trained professionals were saying, "Well, I've resolved most of your symptoms (temporarily); there is nothing more that can be done."

Numerous times during treatment Dr. Mozayeni adjusted my medications based on my changing symptoms. Sixteen months into treatment, the inflammation was decreasing enough that my tissue was better able to metabolize the thyroid medication I was taking. He wanted to decrease my thyroid medication dosage. I was vehemently opposed. I had another physician do the same thing a few years earlier with a very poor outcome and I was terrified of the same thing happening.

I was so wrapped up in fear of re-experiencing that event that I could not remember my body was in a different state than those earlier years.

My body was ready for the change. Dr. Mozayeni knew it. But he had to talk me through it. He also changed the process to a more gradual staging so I could ease into the change.

The point is: I had to trust in a power greater than myself. In this case, I had to trust in the power that guided Dr. Mozayeni's judgment. He sees patients like me every single day. He has treatment protocols that are working. His patients are getting better. I had to remember this and trust in his expertise, knowledge, and data analysis. As time progressed, this became much easier for me, especially as I started to feel better. But it was still a milestone for me to trust a medical professional to the depths required.

Another power greater than myself included the friends around me. I learned to accept friends doing things for me, driving me places, letting my employees take more of my workload. They all wanted to help and weren't sure how. When opportunities arose, they gladly chipped in and did what they could. It was another way for them to express their love and support for me. It was a good exercise for me in accepting love and feeling worthwhile of that love.

I also lost friends during my illness and recovery. Really close friends. And it was hard. It is still hard sometimes. I miss some of those people. But I have learned:

- They probably are not good sources of positive and healing energy for me.
- They might have issues of their own that have nothing to do with me, but had they stayed around, their situations might become draining on me and therefore impair my own healing.
- If they weren't willing to find a way to remain friends in this difficult time, then they probably aren't really a good friend and therefore not a good influence on my healing.

Even chronically ill patients can remain friends, especially with one another. A simple card or note in the mail, a text message, a Facebook message or Tweet can brighten anyone's day. Those who are ill know better than anyone else a short comment can make or break a day. It doesn't have to be a meal, or afternoon spent together. It can be coffee for 30-45 minutes. It can be short and sweet.

I also found getting outside of myself and helping others was an important aspect of my healing. I became a power greater than myself by becoming part of a group that is reaching out and connecting and helping others. I could find people who were in worse situations than I was, who were feeling worse than I was. Helping them helped me heal. I found like-minded people, people who also wanted to heal, to move forward, to get to the other side.

Remember, when helping others, it cannot be to your detriment.

A good friend wisely told me, "Just because you <u>can</u> help someone doesn't mean you should." Choose carefully when you can do this. Timing makes the difference.

Having hope was a key element in my healing as well. If I can't visualize myself at the end, completely healed, then I will never make it there. In the middle of a herx, the hope was definitely not as strong. That's why it is important to keep "the big picture" in mind, and not be stuck in the minutiae of the day.

The final aspect of the Spiritual healing for me was God. I believe in a Higher Power whom I choose to call God. I pray to Him, trust in Him, and know He is with me at all times. I know He has a plan. And I know I am not God. I ask to know His will for me and the knowledge and capability to carry that out. I know patients who are very strong Christians and I know patients who are atheists. Believing in God does not determine whether or not you heal. But believing in a power greater than yourself can make the journey easier and simpler.

Cognitive Repair

A year into treatment, I felt a rush of cognitive improvement within a one week period. I had imagined my cognitive assimilation and processing improving gradually, slowly, almost unnoticeably. And maybe that's how it did happen. But my awareness of the change was an event, not a process.

I met with Dr. Mozayeni on a Friday afternoon to discuss writing this book, still in its infancy state. Usually, Friday afternoons were not a good time for me or for him to attempt anything that required much cognitive processing. By Friday, my brain was usually toast. I don't know why I even agreed to such a meeting at this point, but I did.

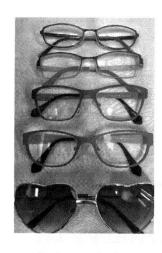

By the end of the two-hour conversation (another first for me in some time), I was still energized and inspired. I wrote. What just transpired was sinking in.

"I haven't felt this "present" in more than a decade. It's been happening over the past two weeks. I keep looking around and seeing the world with a new pair of glasses.

I am starting to be present for conversations, I am literally seeing more clearly, I'm remembering more data and remembering it better. I am working more efficiently.

This is a lot of change. I knew it would get better, but when it gets this much better, it's a tremendous emotional adjustment.

I spent twenty years losing my cognitive abilities, thinking I would never get it back. It is overwhelming and humbling. It's a bit more to take in than I realized.

EMDR helped me realize all the head trash I fed myself to account for my losses.

Whereas Dr. Mozayeni has been able to move forward in incremental steps to make his vision for me come true, I was stuck for two+ decades. I could see the dream, but I couldn't work the steps forward. The energy and mental capabilities are rushing in return.

It's like coming out of anesthesia; I go from pure silence and darkness to the full rush, the sudden WOOSH, of sounds, sights, and sensations in a matter of five seconds.

The physician understands the process. It's data. The physician prescribes the meds; keep the systems in check.

To this patient, it's miraculous and mysterious even when I know the data behind it. And it's very, very emotional.

I trusted Dr. Mozayeni to heal me. I had no idea I would get all this.

I'm getting my life back. I'm getting my dreams back."

Five months later I experienced a similar type of event, though the second one felt even more enhanced. I never took LSD, but somehow, I imagine this experience must be as close to an LSD trip.

Everything was magnified 1000 times. In a one-week time span, I had conversations with people that were more intimate, meaningful, and significant than I had in years before. It was the Aha! conversations where people opened their hearts and souls and secrets to me. I understood the deeper meaning of what my friends were saying to me. I could "take in" what was being said, and process it fully.

In business meetings, I heard what the client was saying, but I also gathered and comprehended any undercurrents to the transaction. I knew what questions to ask to get to the real point.

I sat down to my desk and got my entire To Do List accomplished in a day's time without feeling extreme mental fatigue afterwards.

That was the first week in eight months I had put on makeup and jewelry and came home and fixed dinner for the family.

My writing muse awakened me at 4 am each day, my head filled with poetry and organized thoughts for this book. I wrote for three hours each morning and then went to work each day without an overwhelming sense of fatigue.

"This is the WHOOSH like coming out of anesthesia again that I had in September, only magnified 100 times. I don't know how to process this.

This is like a wave crashing me to ocean floor, crushing the air out of my lungs, swirling debris everywhere around me and I feel every single second magnified by 1000. I swim up for air and pray that it will happen again because it makes me feel alive and engaged.

I am completely overwhelmed in a fantastic way, like trying to pour the ocean into a single glass. Where do I put the rest of it?

Conversations with people are intimate, powerful. I can't drink it in quickly enough. Do I ever get to the point when I can process all this?

Transformational moments I used to get once every few years; I have had five in less than a week.

INTENSE

TRANSFORMING

OVERWHELMING (in a good way)

I don't know how to handle this, how to deal with it. Sitting here unable to write it all down, the feelings are unlanguageable."

Three Phases Create a New Beginning

Most patients who have made it to the end of treatment share a similar experience in that the healing happens in phases and in layers. It is not a neat step-by-step instruction packet. Life's events play a significant role in this process. But our response to those life events is also critical to how we progress (or don't). I still believe the most important components to this part of the healing process are acceptance and willingness.

HOW GOOD
CAN IT GET?

Varying Elements for Healing

Patients vary tremendously in the factors contributing to their condition and symptoms. There is often a much greater range of causal factors than just the *Borrelia burgdorferi* microbe. While there may be other infections that can contribute to the illness, the host response factors are even more varied.

Not only do patients vary, the infections they have vary tremendously and the:

- interplay between the patient,
- their diet and environment,
- their psychological predisposition,
- their financial ability to do what they need to do, and
- the germs they have

will all go into the formula of figuring out not only the time frame but the extent to which a patient can improve.

The patient's support system is also extremely important to the point where it can, potentially, completely negate all of their efforts. As an example, if their spouse is not in alignment with them trying to get better then the patient usually won't get better unless they separate. We have seen this over and over again. Sometimes, as the patient is aligning to heal and they finally find medical support, it could be the precipitant for an already strained relationship to finally break.

Your spouse, your significant other, your family, your workplace, and your other medical care providers all have to be aligned with you.

First, they have to believe you are ill. That is the first step of supporting you. They cannot blame your symptoms on you or some aspect of your personality that makes you come across to them as someone who is not trying or who is complaining or who is whining.

Most people who will have an opinion about your condition are often non-physicians, with no medical expertise, who think somehow they are competent to assess you medically and make conclusions based upon that assessment.

One teacher I treated had a school principal, her boss, tell her she did not have Lyme Disease. This only made the patient more ill.

Typical Improvement

Now, I want to focus on what is typical in terms of patient improvement and healing.

A typical patient who can expect good improvement is someone who may have been sick for years, maybe even decades. I have patients who are finally recovering in their late thirties, who were adolescents or going through puberty when they first became sick. I have seen patients who have fully recovered who have been ill for that long.

It does not appear the duration of your disease determines whether or not you will heal. This is great news for patients who have been ill a long time.

On the other hand, some of these infections over the time frame of a few years or less can cause permanent damage, say to joints. But I haven't seen them cause significant damage to vital organs – at least not in a way we can presently discern.

There are exceptions. *Borrelia* can cause heart block and *Bartonella* can cause heart valve damage (endocarditis), although in the hundreds of patients with *Bartonella* so far, I have not seen it. Except perhaps for some accelerated forms of arthritis in the ankles, knees, and hands, I am not seeing permanent damage. And that is great news.

The typical patient may have been sick for years, if not a decade or more. Because there has been no permanent damage if everything is sorted out and if the right diagnostic, therapeutic, and healing modalities are brought to bear and the patient has the will, the effort, the resources *and* the support then I think the potential for a good outcome is high. That is a lot of "ifs." To put a percentage on it, I would say a patient who has been sick for years, maybe even ten years, could **potentially** get back 90 to 95 percent of the upper limit of their function.

I think it may be more a matter of intensity of effort. No matter how sick you are you really cannot spend your entire day in therapeutic modalities. The practical realistic and often-seen upper limit I think is around 80 to 90 percent. For that reason, the upper limit of healing I mentioned would be reached with simple therapies that are easily maintained – for instance, with some level of support nutritionally, and through the use of supplements and herbs, like broccoli-seed extract, garlic, things that are naturally antimicrobial, naturally anti-inflammatory, and naturally blood thinning in order to help improve the circulation.

Improvement, then, does not necessarily mean a high-maintenance scenario.

If an individual has a strong allergic reaction, an immune reaction, or an inability to detox well from a heavy course of antibiotics that has overburdened their system, this could obviously influence the therapeutic side. For example, some people who have problems with methylation or impairment of other enzymes involved in detoxification, may have a more difficult time with some therapies and may be more dependent on supplements.

Another factor: patients need to be very committed to the process. This can be very difficult. The hardest thing for people to do is to know when they should stop being suspicious of what is being proposed to them. This is a very tough challenge, and it involved – as we said in an earlier chapter – trusting their physician.

There is no way to really guide people who resist your suggested protocol too much. Oftentimes, they perceive the person who is trying to tell them to relax and trust has a potential "conflict of interest" – a patient may believe the practitioner is "trying to push medicines" or is "experimenting" on them. Eventually, the patient has to suspend the disbelief or continue as they have.

At some point patients need to have faith in the process and recognize that it is not perfect. Some things that are tried won't work; that is the nature of healing and healing practices, but it's like trying to find a destination: if you don't try, if you don't seek, for sure, you won't find where it is you need to go.

For physicians, I would say, as long as you know a protocol is safe, it is okay to try new approaches if there is some rational framework. If you have integrity and the patient is also willing to try things and you are both honest about observing what works, then you learn and you can learn quickly. You can really help people heal years before any clinical trial can validate the practice.

The patient needs to be not only in alignment with friends and family but also with the practitioner because it is teamwork for sure.

Spiritual Component

Also, I think there is a huge spiritual component involved in healing from chronic illness. When I see it at work, I am awestruck. I have been personally transformed by seeing how spirituality is transforming and healing for my patients. With these sorts of chronic illnesses, it's like having a flu-like condition for years that's affecting your ability to think and function. It becomes extremely anxiety provoking.

Chronic illness rips people's souls down to the bare bones.

In the process of building themselves back up, I think they all grow tremendously spiritually from it. They don't see the world the same way anymore and their priorities completely shift. This again helps answer the very interesting question: how good can it get?

If you view it properly, in many ways you can actually end up being so much better than you were before you became sick because the processes, the thought patterns, the relationships, that all went into the mix of influences that made you ill have now changed you.

No, I am not saying, "It's all in the patient's head." Not at all. The way we think about things, and the stressors we allow into our lives have a very important role in how our bodies handle pathogens that attack us. People who employ spiritual practices – mind and soul-lifting practices in their healing protocol – can actually end up with a substantial improvement of health because they uncovered and eliminated an unhealthy thought process that gradually caused deterioration which then allowed an acute illness to take hold with the introduction of an infecting pathogen and a dysfunctional host-response.

There is a common theme in almost all of the patients when there was an infectious exposure but there was also a psychosocial stressor (positive or negative), which magnified or accelerated the symptoms.

Mentally it can be a transcending process for them. They can actually be, I think, more enlightened in many ways, more centered, more powerful, and more empowered as a result of recovery from their illness. They also learn a skillset they had not counted on learning. They learn how to preemptively look for and notice these medical problems and deal with them while they are small.

Passing it On

The other thing they can learn in this process is how to teach and mentor others. **The act of trying to help others and heal others is**

in and of itself a healing process, which is one of the reasons why I ultimately arrived at the conclusion that when I am seeing a patient I am not the only healer in the room. In the process of working with patients I found that I receive the healing as well. It's not only the patient. It is a two-way exchange of knowledge, information, emotion, and energy. You have to view it in that way; otherwise, I don't think you can get the full and complete healing you would get. This is true for the patient and practitioner.

In many respects, it is still an exchange.

From the practitioner's point of view it is a hard thing to come in and do every day, to talk to people and carry these emotions. But if you start thinking about it that way it actually becomes more fulfilling and easier. You then deeply feel, not only hear about, the way you have helped people. You can hear about it a lot, you can read about it, but unless you take that positive feedback in and really feel it, it doesn't make you want to keep coming back. It has to be tangible.

Most practitioners who start treating Lyme patients, get busier, faster than they ever imagined because of the demand. They stop accepting new patients or they even stop treating Lyme patients because it is too overwhelming for them. It's like putting their finger into a high-voltage electrical socket at a deep emotional level. Then those practitioners get out.

I wish there was a more formal way to coach physicians who work with chronically ill patients; to support them and develop support groups for them. It is very, very hard. It's not something you aspire to start doing. It is no surprise to me that the medical system typically fails such people and that the core premise that a chronically ill patient can recover is not to be found in the medical system, health insurance process, or society in general.

SHARON

We didn't aspire to be Lyme patients either, but I have seen where the journey takes patients spiritually. For all the pain and exhaustion I have suffered, it has taken me into some mentally, emotionally and spiritually beneficial places.

DR. MOZAYENI

It is critical to develop and maintain a **positive attitude** along the journey. In many ways, you are empowered by it. I am even thinking how we might put patients' experiences to use because they have become real experts at it by the time they are well. They can parlay that into optimizing their future health. They also, then, are in a really good position to help others.

Remission or Cure?

Back on the tangible physical side of the disease, another issue for the patient and physician to analyze carefully is: when is it time to cut back on or end certain treatments?

The problem with all of the microbes we are dealing with is there is no way to prove when you have eradicated them other than by the fact that a patient is feeling well and their inflammation markers are fine, *and* when stressors that could bring back symptoms are gone. This is a functional definition of "cure" rather than a molecular or microbiological definition.

In different fields of medicine physicians are very careful about not using the word "cure." For example, in cancer they will call it a remission not a cure. Sometimes if it has been a good five years past when they might have expected at the least a recurrence they might start calling it a cure. The medical system is very careful to not do that. There are ethical reasons, motivational reasons and also medical-legal reasons behind not pronouncing a patient cured.

If one could kind of put aside those concerns for a minute, we might use the word cure in a more practical sense – which is when a patient can go back to a normal life.

This is possible but patients will want to go to more fulfilling vocations and avocations when they are ready. They rarely want to go back to "who they were" when they became ill.

SHARON

Finding the Balance

Two years (to the day) after I was diagnosed, I wrote:

9:00–10:00 am: Farmer's Market

10:00 am–12:30 pm: blanched kale for green smoothies

12:30–2:00 pm: beginners' yoga

2:30 - 4:00 pm: tea with a newly diagnosed patient

5:30 pm: dinner with Jeff

6:45–7:30 pm: meditation class

8:00 pm: sorting pills for the next two weeks' dosages

AND I AM NOT EXHAUSTED.

A year ago, I could do ONE thing over an entire weekend. I can't believe the improvement. So grateful for an LLMD willing to try new things, for not giving up on me, for helping me HEAL.

The goal is balance. When someone's negative energy comes my way, I have to remember to let it flow THROUGH me, not to soak it up as a sponge and then struggle. I want to keep my balance, keep my grounding as that energy comes and then I want to let it go. I can either be overwhelmed by that negative energy, or I can take it in and then release it with prayers, notes, whatever works for me to disperse it. I cannot ignore that energy, but I do not have to let it consume me and affect my health and well-being.

The same is true for positive energy. When the good stuff comes, I want to accept that energy as it comes to me, but then to let it flow through me. Don't take it all in and let it well up. When that happens, the energy is too much and it exhausts me physically and emotionally. The goal is to accept it and then to let it flowTHROUGH me and out, dispersing in any way I can to others who need it. Like a good dish at the table, "take some and pass it on."

Accepting the New Normal

Three years after starting treatment, I wrote: From the patient perspective of the past two weeks, it's another rocket ship ride. It's a good ride, but it still creates stress. My goal is to accept that this might be the new normal for me.

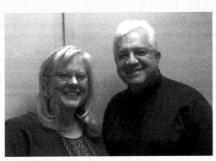

SHARON RAINEY AND BOB MOZAYENI

The difference for me in the energy is that it has filtered down to a cellular level. There is a resurrection of "aliveness" and sensitivity to the living and life I only remember as a young child. I sleep deeply most nights with a sense of revitalization upon waking. I haven't taken a painkiller in two weeks. I can almost work a full day. My passion for writing has become tangible again. I have met friends for lunch and coffee. I am PRESENT for those conversations with friends. I notice the smell of Christmas wreaths. I feel the bite of the cold wind and embrace it instead of shuddering from it. I remember to send bird photos to my friend every day to greet her when she wakes. I can start giving to others and not feel drained.

So much healing has occurred, but it is stressful and different and weird to experience. I must come to this with acceptance and no expectations. This may not be my new normal. It may be a temporary state. I don't know. But I cannot afford to worry about it. I need to accept it and know my body is constantly changing and it's ok. If this is normal, I will adjust to it and accept it. And if it's not, I will find a new balance and equalize with whatever my new normal is.

One practice helping me tremendously is yoga and learning to BREATHE. Sounds crazy, but when I get in the class and they spend ten minutes on breathing, it's amazing how my perspective changes and my equilibrium returns. The meditation is important too.

The important thing is the balance. I have to **not** allow my adrenals go crazy with "HEY YOU FEEL AWESOME! GO DO EVERYTHING YOU CAN RIGHT NOW BEFORE YOU RUN OUT OF ENERGY." Pacing is critical to a pattern of continued healing.

I need not to panic when I wake up at 2 am and can't go back to sleep immediately. It does not mean I am relapsing, it simply means I won't have as good a night's sleep tonight.

I have to stop waiting for the other shoe to drop. It takes time to decondition.

After living with chronic illness for almost three decades, I need to accept my chronic WELLNESS and know I may have a few bumps along the way.

At our first appointment, Dr. Mozayeni saw the person I was supposed to be. I couldn't put that puzzle together like he did at the first meeting. I could see only a fuzzy image at that point. He saw me without the illness. He knew how the illness was affecting me better than I knew.

As the layers have peeled away, I now see what he saw back then. I sold myself short back then, hoping and praying for some of my symptoms to dissipate; I needed the pain to become manageable. I had no idea how sick I was. But he knew. And he saw past it. He knew I could heal. And he knew how life changing the healing would be.

Crossing the Threshold

I remember when my *Bartonella* test results showed no more infection. Dr. Mozayeni said it was ok to stop taking the antibiotics. I sat across from him, shocked, frozen. On one hand, I was elated by the news. I no longer had this horrific disease that had kept me downtrodden for decades. On the other hand, this was all new to me. What was "well" like? How did it feel? What did it look like? I was afraid. And he sensed that.

"Sharon, it's ok. All I have done is open the door for you," he stated. "You can take a step through to the future, or you can simply stand there for as long as you need and take in the view." It took me two more weeks to stop taking the antibiotics. I had to stand there and take in the view. And then – I crossed the threshold, into the healing dimension, into love, into the life I believed could only exist in my dreams.

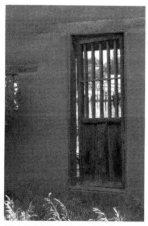

DOOR LEADING FROM A GARDEN WHERE SHARON STAYED IN TAOS, NEW MEXICO. THE VIEW WAS OF THE ENTIRE VALLEY, STUNNING AT SUNSET.

I can't wait for all Lyme patients to see their own initial respective fuzzy image. I can't wait for the image to focus, sharpen, evolve, develop. I can't wait for the healing to begin in them as well. I can't wait for them to find the door, open it, take in the view, and then, to cross the threshold into the dimension of wellness.

SECTION TEN

EXTRA HELP

TANGIBLE TIPS

The following tips are a compilation of suggestions from patients and practitioners. Use the ones you find helpful and forget about the others. Some of these tips contradict one another. That is because different strategies work for different people. We merely want to offer you various options.

SHARON

👥 Doctors' Appointments

- Keep a current hard copy and flash drive list of current meds & supplement list to take with you to doctor's office visits.
- Fill a bag with the stuff you need for your doctor's appointment. Leave it in a place where you won't forget it.
- Ask a friend to go to doctor's appointment with you.
- Bring a lunch, water, and something to comfort you after doctor's appointments.
- Leave time to prepare two days before.

💊 Medications

- Track when you start and stop meds/supplements on calendar.
- Get some small organizing baskets at the dollar store to keep pill bottles in. Also helps make it easier to fill up weekly pills; take baskets right over to the table, sit down and get everything set; so much easier not to fumble with every single bottle.

- Keep med bottles separated so the ones you take on an empty stomach are separate from the ones you take with meals.
- Filling meds & supplements in my pill organizer. Mine is a weekly one divided by Morning, Breakfast, Lunch, Mid-Afternoon, Dinner, and Evening to help me know when to take what and if I have taken it.
- Put your pills out on counter the night before so you see them first thing in the morning.
- Put early a.m. and late p.m. meds by bed with full water bottle.
- Meds can get complicated. Keeping a notepad with meds and writing down what was taken and when will help eliminate the question of "did I take that?"
- Add alarms on your smart phone to remind you when to take your meds.

🍴 Food

- Keep a white board on the fridge so the minute you use something up, you can write it down and it goes on the grocery list.
- Prepare healthy foods in containers (fruit, veggies, salads, etc.) so you can grab them on bad days.
- Soak beans and nuts, have them ready daily for fiber, low gluten meals
- Pre-slice lemons and cucumbers for detox water.
- Squeeze lemons and put in ice trays. Take out cubes of lemon and put in pitcher, add water, sea salt, honey and strawberries.
- Take turmeric or add it to your diet.

- Cook large meals when you are feeling well and freeze for quick reheat when not feeling well.
- Remove sugar from the kitchen.
- Use Corningware instead of stoneware to reduce weight of dishes you have to lift.

🏠 While at Home

- Put things in designated places to reduce frustration
- Keep things in easy to reach places
- Get a grabber - www.ebay.com/bhp/grabber-tool
- Keep notepads and pens all over the house.
- Use a kindle when turning the pages hurts too much.
- Listen to audio books when you don't have the concentration to read.
- Use closed caption on the TV to reduce noise.
- Wear soft cotton clothing for the most part.
- Buy slip on shoes to wear on days you can't manage bending over to tie.
- Keep a walker handy- just in case.
- Have Epsom salts on hand for when you are herxing and need to detox.
- Rinse off after you take a detox bath.
- Install grab bars in the bathroom to help you keep your balance.
- Have a raised toilet seat available in case you need it.
- Have all white sheets and towels by the dozen, ready to wash together including an "ick" towel for when you're really messy.

- Get more pillows and be sure they are clean all the time.
- Buy an end-of-the-bed heating pad; they are great for those with peripheral neuropathy.
- Use a heated mattress pad.
- Wrap the bed frame posts in bubble wrap - I constantly broke my toes on them because I didn't realize where they were.
- Put something near the bed to comfort you when you can't sleep.
- Use Frogg cooling towel.
- Get an easy cot to lie on outdoors.

🎗 Leaving the House

- Switch to across the shoulder purses or messenger bags - they don't hurt your hands or shoulders as much and you are less likely to lose your purse that way.
- Keep earplugs in your purse for when noise gets too loud wherever you are.
- Keep sunglasses in your purse for when your eyes are hypersensitive to light.
- Keep baggies of nuts and dried fruit in your purse for quick energizing snacks.
- Put a scarf or sweater in every bag you leave the house with; wear layers for temperature changes due to Lyme-ish hormonal imbalances.
- Use Peltor earmuffs when going anywhere that has more noise than your brain can process.
- It's ok to ride the scooter in the grocery when you need it.

- Bring your own pillow.
- Carry water with you.
- Handicapped placard for when herxing and fatigue are really bad.
- Use GPS and create memory points for all your destinations.
- Have heat packs with you when traveling for aching muscles.
- Carry ginger for nausea (bad motion sickness whether in car or sometimes standing still!).
- Carry sunblock since many antibiotics make us sun sensitive.
- If there's any risk of being stranded or having to possibly stay overnight, definitely bring a baggie of meds/supplements needed for an extra day.
- Cool packs for neck during heat--heat can affect us to the point of being unable to function even fainting.
- Carry a list of medications you are currently taking.

✅ General

- Set up automatic payments online.
- Set up payments to automatically pay at least the minimum balance on each credit card monthly.
- Use reminders on smart phone.
- Put shopping lists on smart phone, so you don't leave list at home.
- Hang reminder pads with pens on doorknobs, so you can write things down.

- Kitchen—low danger items help. Use an electric kettle to boil water (no flame, automatic shutoff).
- Night lights for hallways.
- Nonskid bathmats and tub mats.
- Simplify your makeup routine.
- Simplify everything.
- Keep simplifying everything.
- Live light.
- Take advantage of better days because on bad days, you can't always get out of bed.
- Some days will be horrible. Forgive yourself for not being able to live up to all the things you think you "should" be doing.
- Do what you need to do when you have the small energy bursts. Learn when your best time is to do things.
- Stop doing things for everyone but yourself.
- Drop everything; pick up only what you can.
- Limit phone, social media and email contacts to what you can handle comfortably.
- Create an Emergency Room box or bag with ER clothing that can be ripped off at the door for washing when you get home, including coat and shoes, so you don't bring ER germs into the house. Also include a hard copy of current meds & supplements.
- Take photos of your rashes.

- Find a system that works, really works, to keep track of symptoms DAILY. There are symptom and medicine trackers Apps. (After a month it's sometimes hard to remember how the month felt with Lyme brain.)
- Keep up with dental care.
- Stay hydrated.
- Find grocery stores that deliver.
- Unsubscribe from catalogs.

MISCELLANEOUS AIDS DURING TREATMENT

I used to believe when I got sick, I could go to the doctor, get a prescription, take a pill, and I would be healed of whatever ailment had inhabited my body. I used to believe a holistic approach to health and well-being was a nice thought, a possible avenue, but something that mostly appealed to those "hippies" or those with a lot of money to throw around.

I used to believe organic food was another way to rip off the customer at the checkout line.

And then I got the Lyme Disease diagnosis. Dr. Mozayeni, with his credentials and research strengths, advised me at my second appointment to go "organic." Some of my blood work came back showing I had significant levels of arsenic in my blood.

I completely understand the panic and desperation late stage cancer patients' experience. I found myself willing to try almost anything to see if it would alleviate my pain and fatigue. I believe in traditional medicine and treatment protocols, but I also now believe a holistic approach is the only way to heal from a systemic, chronic disease.

We have gathered a list some patients have found helpful. What worked for some individuals may or may not work for you. And works now may not work six months from now. The point is, if you want to try it, go for it. People are constantly asking me for the "secrets" to healing. There are none. It's a combination of ingredients unique to each patient.

These are items that were simply helpful during the healing process. They are listed alphabetically.

SHARON

Attitude – A positive attitude is a critical element in my recovery. Even when I'm not feeling well, I know it will get better. At the most difficult and fatiguing phase of therapy, I mentioned to Dr. Mozayeni that I was trying to accept "the new normal" of what I thought my life would be like. I was depressed. He paused, and leaned forward a bit, lowering his voice.

"I need you to do something for me," he said softly. I nodded my head.

"I need you to **aim for no less than a complete cure**," he continued. "I *know* I can heal you, but I need *you* to believe that I can heal you." Dr. Mozayeni's words morphed me into the Energizer Bunny, giving me a new mantra to recite each day.

I printed out "I am aiming for no less than a complete cure" and taped the paper above my desk and on my bathroom mirror as a constant reminder of our ultimate goal. Attitude is key in healing.

Caster oil heat pack - One of the most significant possible benefits of castor oil is being a stimulant to the lymph system, improving lymphatic flow and increasing the activity of the cleansing of tissue.

Coconut oil –

Internal use benefits include:

1. cooking as a dairy free replacement to butter.
2. In green smoothies to boost metabolism and reduce inflammation
3. Oil pulling with coconut oil and a drop of oregano oil helps improve gum health
4. Use as a replacement for vegetable oils in any recipe
5. Mixed with catnip, rosemary, or mint essential oils as a natural bug repellent
6. When taken regularly, it can help fight candida
7. Can boost circulation and help those who often feel cold
8. Ingesting coconut oil daily can help with allergy symptoms
9. A tablespoon melted into a cup of warm tea can help soothe a sore throat
10. It can increase absorption of calcium and magnesium
11. Internally as part of the protocol to help re-mineralize teeth
12. To support healthy thyroid function
13. Its anti-inflammatory properties can help lessen arthritis

14. Coconut oil helps digestion and may fight intestinal parasites or yeast

15. A tablespoon taken before each meal can help improve digestion

16. Can be taken in warm ginger tea to sooth heartburn or nausea

External use benefits include:

1. Body lotion – helps relieve eczema, psoriasis and skin sensitivity

2. As a homemade deodorant

3. As eye-makeup remover

4. Topically to kill yeast infections

5. A tiny dab on the hands and then through hair will help relieve dry brittle hair

6. Rubbed on lips as a natural lip balm

7. On feet to fight athlete's foot

8. Rub inside your nose to alleviate allergy symptoms

9. As a natural shave cream and aftershave lotion; again for those with skin sensitivities

10. Can be used to speed healing of fungal infections when taken internally and used externally

11. By itself or with baking soda as a naturally whitening toothpaste

CPAP and BiPAP machines for sleep apnea – This is one of those things that is good to rule out. The difference I felt after getting a BiPAP machine was remarkable. Part of my fatigue was definitely due to sleep apnea. I had the initial sleep study done AT HOME with a device you wear on your head (VERY SIMPLE). My sleep specialist told me the chronically ill patients he sees have a greater incidence of central sleep apnea rather than obstructive sleep apnea. Central sleep apnea occurs because your brain doesn't send proper signals to the muscles that control your breathing. This condition is different from obstructive sleep apnea, in which you can't breathe normally because of upper airway obstruction. Central sleep apnea is less common than obstructive sleep apnea. But I am told by Dr. Mozayeni, who has researched brain blood flow in sleep apnea, that the sleep apnea may be related to small vessel disease from inflammation. The inflammation in small vessels likely disrupts blood flow and injures the neurons of the brainstem controlling respiratory drive and muscle tone. This is likely the connection between chronic illness and sleep apnea - although the exact mechanism has yet to be proven and will likely be shown to be more complicated than we presently think.

Deep Breathing - When experiencing these vital revelations about the mind body connection, everything seemed exponentially magnified in intensity of light, sound, and touch. I felt like I was on a rocket ship with no space suit; trying to hang on for dear life. The intensity was at times overwhelming for me. I had some difficulty handling the intensity of emotions and thoughts coming through me. My EMDR therapist helped me calm my body and my breath. It slowed the information assimilation and processing for me. It's called 478 breath - www.drweilonhealthyaging.com/hya/ecs/a/video.html

Detox baths – I don't know how much they help medicinally, but it is a good time for me to meditate, relax, and soak up some positive energy. Make sure to rinse everything off after a detox bath!

Dry brushing – (www.iherb.com/Earth-Therapeutics-Massage-Brush/21480?at=0) Dry-brushing is supposed to help with the detoxing process. It helped my skin hypersensitivity and intense itching during herxes. Dry brushing exfoliates dead skin. Since dry skin brushing increases the circulation to the skin, it encourages your body's natural discharge of wastes especially aiding drainage of your lymphatic system whose job it is to remove toxins from the blood and other vital tissues. Treating your skin in this way can also eliminate clogged pores and help your skin to absorb nutrients while aiding in proper excretion of metabolic wastes. Additionally, nerve endings in the skin also become stimulated and help to rejuvenate your nervous system.

eReader (Nook / Kindle / iPad) – at one point, I could not turn the pages of the book because my thumb joints were so painful. An electronic reader allows me to highlight, carry many books at once, and not have to turn pages in a box small enough to fit in my purse.

Crab Bars – My husband installed handicap grab bars for me in the bathroom. The shower was one of the most dangerous places for me. I had trouble keeping my balance while standing, so having the grab bar to hang onto was reassuring. I often didn't pick up my feet enough to get over the tub rim (due to peripheral neuropathy) and can trip too easily. By hanging onto the grab bars, even if I don't pick my foot up enough, I can prevent a bad fall.

Grabber – (www.amazon.com/Ettore-49036-Grip-n-Grab/dp/B001B13PC2/ref=sr_1_1?ie=UTF8&qid=1453922855&sr=8-1&keywords=grabber) or (www.amazon.com/Duro-Med-Aluminum-Reacher-Grabber-Magnetic/dp/B0009STNME/ref=sr_1_4?ie=UTF8&qid=1453922855&sr=8-4&keywords=grabber) - I call it the Grabber. Lower back pain often makes bending over for anything painful. I use the Grabber for picking up anything and everything. It's also good for reaching behind the dryer for those elusive single socks.

Green smoothies and the Vitamix (www.vitamix.com) – My Lymie friend Dan told me he was drinking green smoothies in the morning; they were making a significant difference in his energy levels and were supposedly helpful with reducing inflammation. I said, "If it doesn't taste good, I don't eat or drink it." Dan gave me the recipe, and Jeff bought me the Green Smoothie Revolution (www.amazon.com/Green-Smoothie-Revolution-Radical-Natural/dp/1556438125) book for more recipes. I also found it helpful with reducing my chocolate cravings. My favorite green for the smoothies: kale. Yes, you need the Vitamix in order to do it right. It will make all the difference. I have also heard the Ninja Ultima is a good alternative to the Vitamix (www.ninjakitchen.com/ninja-ultima-blender).

Heating pad for end of the bed – (http://cozywinters.com/shop/bed-foot-warmer.html) Helps keep my feet warm in the winter – **especially important for peripheral neuropathy patients**. It is different than a regular heating pad and better! One can also use an infrared lamp similar to ones used by acupuncturists.

Hobbies – I did a lot of reading during treatment, and not only about Lyme Disease. I read for FUN. It took my mind off reality. For many months, brain fog prevented me from reading anything 'significant.' So the lighter material made it easier to maintain this hobby. I was already an avid knitter and needlepointer; I had to give them up for awhile because the repetitive motion aggravated my joints, but I picked up projects whenever my body allowed.

Hot tub – Jeff liked it for helping to relax his muscles, a good time and place for meditation as well. If you have skin issues, be careful, as chemicals can sometimes irritate. The bromine may compete with iodine in your system so be sure your iodine intake is adequate.

Intuition – Listen to it; follow your gut.

Laughter - Hours and hours of "Whose Line is it Anyway?" and

"Big Bang Theory" worked best for me. Laughter heals. When I asked fellow Lymies for their suggestions for this list of practical aids, many of them stated, "Laughter is the most important." Numerous studies have shown laughter releases endorphins. And that can only make one feel better.

Meal planning – A game changer for me was signing up for the monthly program of nutrition counseling and meal planning at www.chroniclymenutrition.com. Creator and owner Robin Shirley provides a full meal plan and schedule and even the shopping list. She explains why it's important to eat various foods and how they can impact the healing process. Robin took the thinking out of food preparation for me and I sorely needed this. Her program does much more than simple meal planning, but that was the big attraction for me.

Meditation – I still struggle with this one. I have tried many different types of meditation, some more successful than others. My "mantra" to you is to keep trying until you find something that works. And some types may work for a while and then you may need to adjust. The important aspect of this is to find a way to get your body and mind quiet for a period of time each day.

Naps – I take them often. NOT taking a nap was detrimental to my health. Rest is an essential part of the healing process. I cannot emphasize this enough.

Nutritionist – Initially, I only needed a few sessions with a nutritionist after Dr. Mozayeni's suggestion to go gluten and dairy free. Eliminating gluten and dairy products significantly improved my intestinal tract problems. I needed help from a nutritionist to show me options and alternatives. She taught me how to make toasted kale disguised as potato chips. She introduced me to dehydrated bread. She also took me through a few grocery stores to familiarize me with healthier options. I still need more sessions with a nutritionist to get me through the "no sugar" portion of my life - one step at a time.

Personal Trainer – It was almost two years into treatment before I could do any sort of exercise. When I re-started, I was terrified of re-injuring myself. I found a trainer who was previously a US Army Master Fitness Trainer. She helped injured servicemen regain full physical mobility. It's important to find the right match and to find someone who is educated and experienced so they don't let you injure yourself.

Pill Boxes – (www.amazon.com/Compartment-Pill-Organizer-DEEP-

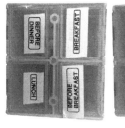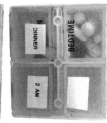

Inch/dp/B000E13BVA) I used these, making my own label for each section: Before Breakfast, Breakfast, Before Lunch, Lunch, Before Dinner, Dinner, Bedtime, 2 AM. So I needed two boxes for each day. The 1-inch deep ones were big enough to hold all of my pills. I took approximately 40-50 pills daily during treatment.

Progress Journal - In a simple Excel spreadsheet, I recorded the date and the event of anything significant for me. I referred back to this spreadsheet often, especially during herxes, to remind me of the progress I had made. I included things like "made the bed," "started putting on make up," and "shaved my legs 5 days in a row."

Rest – I cannot emphasize this enough. I live in an area of the country where "downtime" is not encouraged. And this was probably the most difficult element for me to maintain during my treatment. I am convinced rest is an essential part of my recovery. Notice I wrote "Naps" and "Rest" as two separate items. That is because they <u>are</u> two separate items. You need BOTH. And they are ESSENTIAL to HEALING.

Soap – My skin started reacting to almost anything I put on my skin. I stopped wearing makeup. I had to find a soap that didn't cause more skin breakouts. I use fragrance free unscented soap and haven't had an issue since I started using it. As I have healed, I have started being able to tolerate some soap with essential oils included. I get those from I get those from <u>www.etsy.com/shop/BadRickSoaps</u>.

Stick with the Winners – Connecting with others who have the same disease is a huge aid during treatment. It is important to choose those "others" carefully. Staying positive is a key element of a successful recovery. I chose to surround myself with those who exuded compassion, genuine positive energy, humor, and fierce determination. We fed off of each other's energy throughout our respective treatments.

Stretching – (www.simplefitnesssolutions.com/stretch.htm). I stretch in bed before I get up, I stretch sitting on the bed, standing in the shower, drying my hair, putting on my clothes. I stretch in my chair at work, on the couch at home. I stretch whenever and wherever possible. The strap is helpful when muscles are really tight.

Trigger Point Injections – I received trigger point injections of Marcaine and Toradol. These are NOT steroids. Toradol is an anti-inflammatory. Marcaine is local anesthetic. These injections gave me short periods of being pain free, something I had not experienced in decades. I had no idea the exhaustion chronic pain causes until I had none for those 24 hours.

After the first two injections, I got up from the exam table and realized I had moved from a prone position to standing up without any pain. The smile that grew across my face was the size of the Cheshire cat's. I leaned over to pick up my jeans, bending straight and forward, no favoring of either side. I giggled. I stepped each leg into the jeans easily. More giggling. I bent over and picked up my sneakers. It felt as though I had "gotten away with something."

Dr. Mozayeni came back into the room and asked, "How do you feel?"

I sat in the chair and lifted my right leg with absolutely no pain. I repeatedly stood up and sat down, straight and balanced with no hesitation. When standing, I bent over and touched the floor with my hands, again, with no jerky movement, and absolutely no pain.

Completely overwhelmed with gratitude and excitement, I could only utter, "This is mondo-bizarro." Dr. Mozayeni chuckled in retort. I walked out of his office looking like the cat that ate the canary. I did not stop smiling for the rest of the evening.

Most of the above are items I never would have considered before my illness. But when we want to heal, willingness becomes key in our attempt to find what works and what will keep us on the path to healing. I found many of the above items helpful in my recovery. I hope you do as well.

Meditation:

- *Passage Meditation* by Eknath Easwaran
- *Conquest of the Mind* by Eknath Easwaran
- *Embracing Healing – a Slow Down Thirty Day Practice* by Christina Murphy, CHC, AADP

Mind Body Connection, Energy, Energy Fields, Mind-over Matter:

- *The Intention Experiment* by Lynne McTaggart
- *The Field* by Lynne McTaggart
- *The Biology of Belief* by Bruce H. Lipton, Ph.D.
- *Earthing: The Most Important Health Discovery Ever!* by Clinton Ober
- *Positive Energy* by Judith Orloff, MD
- *Power vs. Force* by David Hawkings, MD
- *Healing and Recovery* by David Hawkings, MD

Spiritual & Consciousness Based:

- *The Power of Now* by Eckhart Tolle
- *A New World* by Eckhart Tolle
- *The Seat of the Soul* by Gary Zukav
- *Conversations with God* by Neale Donald Walsch
- *Many Lives Many Masters* by Brian Weiss, MD

- *Awakening into ONENESS* by Arjuna Ardagh
- *The Alchemist* by Paulo Coelho
- *Blink* by Malcolm Gladwell
- *The Invitation* by Oriah Mountain Dancer

Religious:

- *Autobiography of a Yogi* by Paramhansa Yogananda
- *The World's Religions* by Huston Smith

Buddhist Teachings:

- *Essence of the Heart Sutra* by The Dalai Lama
- *The Essence of Happiness* by The Dalai Lama

Philosophy, Psychology and Self Help:

- *365 Prescriptions for the Soul: Daily Messages of Inspiration, Hope, and Love* by Dr. Bernie Siegel
- *A Mile in My Shoes* by Trevor Hudson
- *A Return to Love* by Marianne Williams
- *The Best Part of My Day Healing Journal* by Sharon E. Rainey
- *Carry On, Warrior: The Power of Embracing Your Messy, Beautiful Life* by Glennon Doyle Melton
- *The Four Agreements* by Don Miguel Ruiz
- *How to Heal Yourself When No One Else Can* by Amy B. Scher
- *The Last Best Cure: My Quest to Awaken the Healing Parts of My Brain and Get Back My Body, My Joy and My Life* by Donna Jackson Nakazawa

- *Learned Optimism* by Martin E. Seligman, Ph.D.
- *Loving What Is* by Byron Katie
- *Soul Repair: Rebuilding Your Spiritual Life* by Jeff VanVonderen

Directly Lyme Related:

- *A Twist of Lyme: Battling a Disease that "Doesn't Exist"* by Andrea Caeser
- *Autoimmune Illness and Lyme Disease Recovery* by Katina I. Makris
- *Beyond* Lyme Disease*: Healing the Underlying Causes of Chronic Illness in People with Borreliosis and Co-Infections* by Connie Strasheim and Lee Cowden MD
- *Chronic Illness as an Access to Quantum Healing* by Jenny Rush
- *Coping with* Lyme Disease*: A Practical Guide to Dealing with Diagnosis and Treatment* by Denise Lang and Kenneth Liegner
- *Cure Unknown: Inside the Lyme Epidemic* by Pamela Weintraub
- *Gone in a Heartbeat – A Physician's Search for True Healing* by Neil Spector, MD
- *"It's All In Your Head", Around the World in 80 Lyme Patient Stories: Valid Reasons to Debate Current Treatment* by PJ Langhoff
- *Nature's Dirty Needle: What You Need to Know About Chronic* Lyme Disease *and How to Get the Help To Feel Better* by Mara Williams
- *Out Of The Woods: Healing* Lyme Disease *Body, Mind & Spirit*

by Katina Makris

- *The Beginner's Guide to Lyme Disease: Diagnosis and Treatment Made Simple* by Nicola McFadzean N.D. and Joseph J. Burrascano Jr. M.D.
- *If I Only Had a Brain Injury: A TBI Survivor and Life Coach's Guide to Chronic Fatigue, Concussion, Lyme Disease, Migraine or Other "Medical Mystery"* by Laura Bruno

Medical and Trauma Related:

- *The Anatomy of Hope* by Jerome Groopman
- *Hypothyroidism Type 2: The Epidemic* by Mark Starr
- *Invisible Heroes – Survivors of Trauma and How They Heal* by Belleruth Naparstek
- *The Trauma Spectrum: Hidden Wounds and Human Resiliency* by Robert C. Scaer
- *Waking the Tiger: Healing Trauma: The Innate Capacity to Transform Overwhelming Experiences* by Peter A. Levine, Ann Frederick

Films

The Living Matrix

What the Bleep Do We Know (2004)

Ram Dass Fierce Grace (2001)

Conversations with God (2006)

Under Our Skin (2009)

Under Our Skin – Part 2: Emergence (2015)

Websites

- Chronic Lyme Nutrition – www.chroniclymenutrition.com

- Galaxy Diagnostics - www.galaxydx.com

- International Lyme and Associated Diseases Society (ILADS) – www.ilads.org

- Beating *Bartonella* - www.beating*Bartonella*.com

- Fisher Wallace Laboratories - www.fisherwallace.com

- What is Lyme? - www.whatislyme.comweb.ncsu.edu

- Translational Medicine Group - www.tmgmd.com

- Better Health Guy - www.betterhealthguy.com

- Lyme Disease.org - www.lymedisease.org

- National Capital Lyme Disease Association - www.natcaplyme.org

- www.lymenet.org

- www.lymediseaseassociation.org

- www.publichealthalert.org

- www.lymeinfo.net

- www.lymefriends.org

- www.lymepedia.org

- www.lymediseaseaudio.com

- www.underourskin.com

- www.lymepa.org

- www.lymetap.org

- www.ceresnano.com/nanotrap-lyme-test

- www.sharonrainey.com

Blogs

- But You Don't Look Sick - www.butyoudontlooksick.com

- Chronically Living - slippingthroughthecracks.blogspot.com

- Lady of Lyme - www.ladyoflyme.com

- Lyme and a Coconut - https://lymeandacoconut.wordpress.com

- Lyme Chick blog - www.lymechick.com

- Lyme Disease Resource - lymediseaseresource.com/wordpress

- Lyme Savvy – www.lymesavvy.com

- Overcoming Lyme - overcominglyme.blogspot.com

- Wild Condor - www.wildcondor.com

- LifeLoveLyme - lifelovelyme.com

- Will There Be Cake? - willtherebecake.org

ACKNOWLEDGEMENTS

"Gratitude unlocks the fullness of life. It turns what we have into enough, and more. It turns denial into acceptance, chaos to order, confusion to clarity. It can turn a meal into a feast, a house into a home, a stranger into a friend, gratitude makes sense of our past, brings peace for today, and creates a vision for tomorrow."

– MELODIE BEATTIE

Troup Brazelton – those fateful words led me to the path of healing: "You don't have Lupus, you have Lyme." You saved my life; **Terrill Brazelton** – I remember when you told me about the dream you had right after your mom died. She came to you and said it was going to be all right. That doesn't make your pain any less. She really is all right. I hear her laughing when I walk by the woods next to our house. I felt her when I was writing parts of this book. Your mother and father are IN this book. **Nichole Rodriguez** started it again with "you have to see my boss's Lyme doctor;" **Dolores Bowen** - for your hours and hours and hours of transcribing Dr. M's and my interviews. This book would never have happened without your time and talent; **Reuben Jackson** – who kept saying, "You'll be alright." And you were right. Thanks for keeping the faith with me, thanks for grieving with me and helping me heal, thank you for letting me keep three lines in each poem; **Deb Jansen** – for giving me the pen and the courage to use it, your hysterical one liners, your willingness to sit through "Big Bang Theory" with me night after night after night, and most of all, thank you for letting me love you; **Dan Frumkin** – for repeatedly connecting with me and sharing every piece of information – the good, the bad, and the ugly. You were the first one to offer me hope of healing; **Mary B** – for staying connected with me, your depth, your humor, your insights and feedback, your tenacity; **Lisa Hilton** – from Day 1 you encouraged me to write this book. Thank you for your faith in me; **Representative Barbara Comstock** was the Chief Patron of the "Lyme Disease Information

SHARON

Disclosure Act" which passed the Virginia General Assembly. This bill allows Virginians to be educated and informed of the limitations of the existing serologic tests currently used to detect Lyme Disease and the problem of false negatives in these tests; Barbara is now my U.S. Congressional representative and more importantly, my friend; **Amanda Elam** – my "voice of reason;" **Alyssa Knapp** – long distance friendship can work when the souls are so similar; **Nullie Stockton** – one of my Earth angels who surprises me with healing foods and healing laughter; **Gary Glaser** – Rest in Peace, my friend. Lyme took you too soon; my readers **Matt Jablow, Rhonda Sheehan, Angela Castle, Ruth James, Deb Kushner, and Heather Solano** – your honesty, fresh view, and frank dialogue were life savers to me in my time of doubt; **to the hundreds of Lyme patients who met me for coffee, Facebooked me, Tweeted me, and rallied with me** – thank you for entrusting me with your stories, your fears and your fights. Each one of you is in this book. I wrote with you in mind, what you wanted me to say for you, what you need to hear, what you want to read. We WILL heal. We WILL conquer this disease; **Heather Rainey** – for being my sugar sponsor, for leading me to healthy eating and healthy living, and for reconnecting with love and acceptance. I love you, Heather; **Cindy Murphy** – for being my first reader (and incredible editor), my smoothie maker, my front row cheerleader; the first to take my call when Riley was killed; my Santa Fe sanity; **Kathy Pesavento** – for introducing me to trigger point release therapy, and yes, even to dry needling. Thank you for never giving up on my healing; **Kathryn Ford** – I never would have made it to the other side without your professional talent and compassion; **Beth Renne** – thank you for opening the door and shining the light; **Joanne Muir** – you see me at my most vulnerable and you hold that space sacred for me - thank you; **Patricia Nwanz** – your skill in your profession lessens my anxiety and helps me heal; **Tami Griffin** – thank you for every time you have sat beside me in silence, holding my hand, praying with me; **Ed Breitschwerdt** for your compassion, continued dedication, and sheer brilliance; you are still a rock star to me; **Stephen Xenakis** – your no-nonsense approach and your quiet compassion are just the right mix; thank you for saving my sanity, and those around me; **Riley Rainey** – my healing buddy, you were in my life for too little time. Thank you for opening my heart and filling it with sheer joy and innocence; **Suzanne Mozayeni** – for opening your heart and spirit; **Mom and Dad (Earle and June Williams)** – your generous support (financial and emotional) afforded Jeff, Stephen, and me the opportunity to heal from these treacherous infections; my gratitude will never be adequately expressed in proportion to the emotion attached to it; I hope this book will help others to find healing so they will not suffer the same tragedy as Aunt Betty did; you play a key role in that change; as a result, your support of my healing is responsible for the healing of thousands more who follow; you are leaving a legacy of healing for so many; **Stephen Anson Rainey** – your healing was a tremendous role model as I followed behind. Thank you for your constant encouragement and for reminding your mother that the healing is just around the corner. Thank you for being comfortable in silence, for your sensitivity. You are indeed, an old soul; **Jeffrey Allen Rainey** – no one will know the depth of sacrifices you made for decades (and still make) while I suffered through these illnesses and then healed; no one will know how often you rubbed my painful joints, held me in the middle of the night as I sobbed with pain and fear and anxiety; but I know. You stayed with a very sick woman. You took your marriage vows solemnly, having no idea how deeply and broadly you would be tested. You helped me heal from the cellular level with unbridled and unending love, dedication, optimism, an organic garden, raw and unfiltered honey, and still even more love. I love you, Jeffrey, to infinity and beyond. – SER

DR. MOZAYENI

First and foremost, I wish to acknowledge the patients who encouraged me constantly to persevere in helping them - by showing me their determination, diligence and courage to endure their suffering one day at a time. My job is to know as much as I can, learning as much as possible from every patient encounter so I may help the next patient more effectively.

This process is grueling for patients, but it is also grueling for practitioners genuinely committed to helping find solutions in a 'system' of health care that dissuades regularly, obstructs often, and punishes occasionally a new thought no matter how logical or obvious the underlying medical science may be.

To delay gratification, an individual needs to have had the love of parents and then, his own family, to be able to persevere in difficult pursuits. I have had both.

Knowledge through training and experience is important, but the ability to think clearly and compassionately is something one picks up from excellent mentors – teachers who empower you, helping you grow, gain confidence in your learning, and professionally execute your knowledge and talent. I have had many excellent mentors and we all have a responsibility to pass this on to others.

An important part of the equation in the doctor-patient relationship is to have mutual concern and respect – I hope patients feel more empowered and enabled from the first minute of our first appointment. In turn, and I hope a patients help their doctor feel good about the work s/he is doing and once in a while, send an uplifting note of encouragement to that physician, especially when they recognize the potential for burnout. Many of my patients have sent me such messages exactly when needed. I am grateful to each of them them for appreciating the effort - we appreciate one another.

I could list many names as is customary in acknowledgements. But you know who you are and so do I.

Then, on the other hand, there are also those rare patients who are in such extreme turmoil in their own lives that they have no idea how much emotional harm they do to others in their actions. They harm not only themselves, but also others - and they harm other patients by occasionally forcing us practitioners put up our defenses and shut down our compassion for other patients. We must acknowledge these patients too, as they know not what they do and provide wonderful contrast with which we can appreciate the angels among our patients and remember why we do this hard work.

It is also important to acknowledge the practitioners who turn away from the chronically ill with all sorts of excuses - there is no 'evidence' or it is 'all in their head'. You have provided the negative example and contrast against which the work of compassionate doctors is valued. History in general, and medicine in particular, is full of people who say it can't be done. It's ok if you don't want to try or can't try, but please do not get in the way of those who do try because, one day, you will need someone to try to help you.

I hope this book will provide doctors and patients alike some insights into the psycho-social dynamic of the doctor-patient relationship that is needed to help with the recovery from chronic illness. Every patient who recovers from chronic illness teaches those who don't believe they are sick much needed compassion for those who suffer alone quietly with no obvious outward evidence of illness. Later, in witnessing the recovery of these patients, we are all empowered because we witness what is possible and it gives us all hope.

The recovery of every chronically ill patient has a far-reaching positive impact on all of us. The net result: patients and practitioners alike are forever transformed.   – BRM

GLOSSARY

Abx - Sometimes you will see the word antibiotics shortened to "abx."

***Bartonella* -** a genus of Gram-negative bacteria. Facultative intracellular parasites, *Bartonella* species can infect healthy people but are considered especially important as opportunistic pathogens. *Bartonella* are transmitted by insect vectors such as ticks, fleas, sand flies, and mosquitoes.

Bayesian probability decision-making - a probability system that tries to quantify the tradeoff between various decisions, making use of probabilities and costs. An agent operating under such a decision theory uses the concepts of Bayesian probability models to estimate the expected value of its actions, and update its expectations based on new information.

***Borrelia burgdorferi* -** a bacterial species of the spirochete class of the genus *Borrelia*.

The causative agent is named after the researcher Willy Burgdorfer, who first isolated the bacterium in 1982.

Citizen science - scientific research conducted, in whole or in part, by amateur or nonprofessional scientists, often by crowdsourcing and crowd funding. Formally, citizen science has been defined as "the systematic collection and analysis of data; development of technology; testing of natural phenomena; and the dissemination of these activities by researchers on a primarily avocational basis". Citizen science is sometimes called "public participation in scientific research."

EIA test - The first part of a two-step process when testing blood for evidence of antibodies against the Lyme Disease bacteria. If the "EIA" (enzyme immunoassay) or rarely, an "IFA" (indirect immunofluorescence assay) is negative, no further testing of the specimen is usually done. If the first step is positive or indeterminate (sometimes called "equivocal"), the second step is performed. The second step uses a test called an immunoblot test, commonly, a "Western blot" test. Results are considered positive only if the EIA/IFA and the immunoblot are both positive.

Heme - the deep red, nonprotein, ferrous component of hemoglobin.

Herxheimer or "herx" – The Jarisch-Herxheimer reaction is a short-term (from days to a few weeks) detoxification reaction in the body. As the body detoxifies, it is not uncommon to experience flu-like symptoms including headache, joint and muscle pain, body aches, sore throat, general malaise, sweating, chills, nausea or other symptoms.

This is a normal reaction indicating parasites, fungus, viruses, bacteria or other pathogens are being effectively killed off. The biggest problem with the Herxheimer reaction is people stop taking the supplement or medication causing the reaction, and thus discontinue the very treatment helping to make them better. Although the experience may not make you feel particularly good, the Herxheimer Reaction is actually a sign that healing is taking place. The Herxheimer Reaction is an immune system reaction to the toxins (endotoxins) that are released when large amounts of pathogens are being killed off, and the body does not eliminate the toxins quickly enough. It is a reaction occurring when the body is detoxifying and the released toxins either exacerbate the symptoms being treated or create their own symptoms. The important thing to note is worsening symptoms do not indicate failure of the treatment in question; in fact, usually the opposite. The most common terminology used is the Herxheimer Reaction. It is also often referred to as a healing crisis, a detox reaction, or die-off syndrome.

IgG and IgM - two types of antibodies found in the blood. Antibodies are part of the body's immune system used to identify, neutralize, and destroy foreign objects and organisms, such as bacteria, parasites, and viruses. At a basic level, IgM antibodies usually are associated with the early onset phase of an infection (acute), while IgG is generally associated with long-term immunity or reactivity towards a pathogen (chronic).

myelin – an electrical stimulating material that forms a layer, the **myelin sheath**, usually around only the axon of a neuron. It is essential for the proper functioning of the nervous system.

Occam's razor or Ockham's razor - a principle of economy or succinctness used in logic and problem-solving. It states that among competing hypotheses, the hypothesis with the fewest assumptions should be selected. The application of the principle often shifts the burden of proof in a discussion. The razor states one should proceed to simpler theories until simplicity can be traded for greater explanatory power. The simplest available theory need not be most accurate. Philosophers also point out the exact meaning of *simplest* may be nuanced. In science, Occam's razor is used as a heuristic (general guiding rule or an observation) to guide scientists in the development of theoretical models rather than as an arbiter between published models.

Off-label - Off-label use is the use of pharmaceutical drugs or devices in a way that has not had a marketing claim approved by the FDA for an unapproved indication or in an unapproved age group, unapproved dosage, or unapproved form of administration. Both prescription drugs and over-the-counter drugs (OTCs) can be used in off-label ways, although most study of off-label use centers on prescription drugs. Off-label use is generally legal unless it violates specific ethical guidelines or safety regulations, but it does carry health risks and differences in legal liability. Physicians, under state licenses, are permitted to prescribe "off-label".

One Health Initiative – The One Health Initiative is a movement to forge co-equal, all inclusive collaborations between physicians, osteopaths, veterinarians, dentists, nurses and other scientific-health and environmentally related disciplines. Recognizing that human health (including mental health via the human-animal bond phenomenon), animal health, and ecosystem health are inextricably linked, One Health seeks to promote, improve, and defend the health and well-being of all species by enhancing cooperation and collaboration between physicians, veterinarians, other scientific health and environmental professionals and by promoting strengths in leadership and management to achieve these goals. One Health is dedicated to improving the lives of all species—human and animal—through the integration of human medicine, veterinary medicine and environmental science. This shall be achieved through joint educational efforts between human medical, veterinary medical schools, and schools of public health and the environment; joint communication efforts in journals, at conferences, and via allied health networks; joint efforts in clinical care through the assessment, treatment and prevention of cross-species disease transmission; joint cross-species disease surveillance and control efforts in public health; joint efforts in better understanding of cross-species disease transmission through comparative medicine and environmental research; joint efforts in the development and evaluation of new diagnostic methods, medicines and vaccines for the prevention and control of diseases across species and; joint efforts to inform and educate political leaders and the public sector through accurate media publications.

PANDAS - Pediatric Autoimmune Neuropsychiatric Disorders Associated with Streptococcal infections, a disease in which a subset of children are thought to exhibit a rapid onset of obsessive-compulsive disorder (OCD) and/or tic disorders symptoms following group A beta-hemolytic streptococcal (GABHS) infections. The proposed link between infection and these disorders is an initial autoimmune reaction to a GABHS infection producing antibodies, continuing to interfere with basal ganglia function, causing symptom exacerbations. Obsessive Compulsive Disorder (OCD) and/or tic disorders suddenly appear following a strep infection (such as strep throat or scarlet fever); or the symptoms of OCD or tic symptoms suddenly become worse following a strep infection. The symptoms are usually dramatic, happen "overnight and out of the blue," and can include motor and/or vocal tics, obsessions, and/or compulsions. In addition to these symptoms, children may also become moody, irritable, experience anxiety attacks, or show concerns about separating from parents or loved ones.

PCR tests or Polymerase Chain Reaction - a technique used to amplify very small amounts of DNA to detectable levels. This allows extremely sensitive detection of pathogens. If a positive detection is suspected, the organism is sequenced and the exact species identified.

Protozoan infections - *Protozoan* infections are single-cell parasitic diseases organisms formally classified in the Kingdom Protozoa.

They include organisms classified in Amoebozoa, Excavata, and Chromalveolata. Examples include *Entamoeba histolytica*, *Plasmodium* (some of which cause malaria), *Babesia* and *Giardia lamblia. Trypanosoma brucei*, transmitted by the tsetse fly and the cause of African sleeping sickness, is another example. The species traditionally collectively termed "*Protozoa*" are not closely related to each other, and have only superficial similarities (eukaryotic, unicellular, motile, though with exceptions.) The terms "*Protozoa*" (and protist) are usually discouraged in the modern biosciences. However, this terminology is still encountered in medicine. This is partially because of the conservative character of medical classification, and partially due to the necessity of making identifications of organisms based upon appearances and not upon DNA.

Quorum Sensing - a system of stimulus and response correlated to population density. Many species of bacteria use quorum sensing to coordinate gene expression according to the density of their local population. Quorum sensing can function as a decision-making process in any decentralized system, as long as individual components have: (a) a means of assessing the number of other components they interact with and (b) a standard response once a threshold number of components is detected. Bacteria that use quorum sensing constitutively produce and secrete certain signaling molecules (called *auto inducers* or *pheromones*). These bacteria also have a receptor that can specifically detect the signaling molecule (inducer). When the inducer binds the receptor, it activates transcription of certain genes, including those for inducer synthesis. In order for gene transcription to be activated, the cell must encounter signaling molecules secreted by other cells in its environment. When only a few other bacteria of the same kind are in the vicinity, diffusion reduces the concentration of the inducer in the surrounding medium to almost zero, so the bacteria produce little inducer. However, as the population grows, the concentration of the inducer passes a threshold, causing more inducer to be synthesized. This forms a positive feedback loop, and the receptor becomes fully activated.

Spirochete - The shape and class *Borrelia* is in. Under a microscope this bacteria looks like a corkscrew.

Translational medicine (also referred to as translational science) is a discipline within biomedical and public health research aiming to improve the health of individuals and the community by "translating" findings into diagnostic tools, medicines, procedures, policies and education. Translational medicine is a rapidly growing discipline in biomedical research and aims to expedite the discovery of new diagnostic tools and treatments by using a multi-disciplinary, highly collaborate, "bench-to-bedside" approach. Within public health, translational medicine is focused on ensuring proven strategies for disease treatment and prevention are actually implemented within the community. One prevalent description of translational medicine, first introduced by the Institute of Medicine's Clinical Research Roundtable, highlights two roadblocks (i.e., distinct areas in need of improvement): the first translational block (T1) prevents basic research findings from being tested in a clinical setting; the second translational block (T2) prevents proven interventions from becoming standard practice.

Vector Borne Disease – an illness caused by an infectious microbe transmitted to people by blood-sucking arthropods. The arthropods (insects or arachnids) most commonly serving as vectors include: blood sucking insects such as mosquitoes, fleas, lice, biting flies and bugs, and blood sucking arachnids such as mites and ticks. The term "vector" refers to any arthropod transmitting a disease through feeding activity. Vectors typically become infected by a disease agent while feeding on infected vertebrates (e.g., birds, rodents, other larger animals, or humans), and then pass on the microbe to a susceptible person or other animal. In almost all cases, an infectious microbe must infect and multiply inside the arthropod before the arthropod is able to transmit the disease through its salivary glands.

A practical day-by-day reflection workbook on healing, gratitude and living your best life.

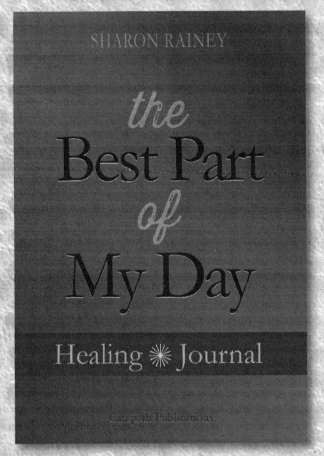

New! A unique resource designed for chronic illness survivors, their caregivers, and anyone seeking a more balanced, thoughtful life.

Written by Sharon Rainey, Lyme Survivor and Advocate, Entrepreneur and Author, this book is the perfect hands-on resource to quickly and easily meditate on and take note of the little things throughout the day that add up to a life of grace and joy.

ORDER TODAY AT
SHARONRAINEY.COM

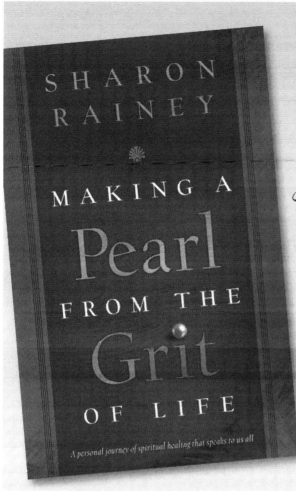

A personal journey of spiritual healing that speaks to us all

"And then something shifted inside me, and I saw how to make my life a blessing..."

"Everyone has interesting, amazing stories; but they very rarely share them in the way that Sharon has"
—ARANYA TOMSETH

"Authentic, transparent, filled with integrity"
—MARY BUSH

"Sharon points a light to the path of healing"
—TONIA VAUGHN

Making a Pearl from the Grit of Life allows us to follow Sharon Rainey on a very private path of early trauma. It leads us through depths of the human spirit - depths we come to recognize as very much like our own - and, through hard-won lessons, emerge onto a higher place of inner strength and happiness.

order today at **www.sharonrainey.com**

Made in the USA
Lexington, KY
19 April 2017